EASY SOMATIC EXERCISES FOR BEGINNERS

28 Days of Somatic Release to Dissolve Tension and Find Peace.

By

Brienne Turner

Table of Content

INTRODUCTION

Somatic exercises are a gentle yet powerful approach that helps foster a harmonious relationship between your mind and body. In this beginner's guide, my goal is to demystify somatics and provide you with a practical roadmap to begin your own journey of self-discovery and well-being.

Somatic exercises enhance your awareness of bodily sensations, promoting relaxation and releasing accumulated tension. For beginners, this means an accessible entry point into mindful movement, where the focus is not just on physical activity but on cultivating a deeper understanding of your body's signals.

In the following pages, I'll explore various somatic exercises, breaking them down into simple steps accompanied by clear images. My goal is to make the practice easily understandable and achievable, ensuring that you can seamlessly incorporate these exercises into your daily routine.

Why engage in somatic exercises? The benefits are subtle yet profound. These exercises offer a gentle approach to improving posture, alleviating discomfort, and enhancing overall physical comfort. They empower you to become more attuned to your body's unique needs, promoting a sense of ease and well-being in your daily life.

As you read through this guide, you'll not only learn the basics of somatic exercises but also find a 28-day plan to kickstart your somatic journey. This plan is designed for anyone, regardless of their fitness level or prior experience, who wants to incorporate somatic practices into their routine and enjoy the benefits of increased body awareness and relaxation.

So, if you're looking for a practical and straightforward way to enter the world of mindful movement, this guide is here to help you.

CHAPTER 1: INTRODUCTION TO SOMATICS

Before we kick things off, I will dedicate this chapter to the "why" and "how" of Somatics, to set up a comfortable spot before the real fun begins. Here, I will help you figure out what these exercises are all about, and why they are so amazing for your soul (even if you're a beginner!).

Understanding Somatic Exercises

Somatics, a holistic approach to understanding and addressing pain, discomfort, and imbalances within the body, emerged in the 1970s through the pioneering work of Thomas Hanna, Ph.D. Hanna conceptualized somatics as a set of movement and relaxation techniques designed to enhance individuals' awareness of their bodies. Building upon this foundation, Peter Levine, Ph.D., later developed a specialized form of therapy known as "somatic experiencing," with a primary focus on assisting people in managing trauma and stress-related disorders.

Somatic therapy, also referred to as somatic experiencing therapy, uniquely integrates mind-body techniques to target both the physical and psychological symptoms associated with various mental health conditions. While it is widely recognized for its effectiveness in trauma treatment, somatic therapy has proven valuable in supporting individuals dealing with a spectrum of issues, including anxiety, depression, grief, anger, trust concerns, and intimacy issues.

Engaging in somatic exercises yields a myriad of mental and physical health benefits. Notably, these exercises are designed to be accessible to individuals of all ages, abilities, and fitness levels, as they are not physically demanding. Moreover, the beauty of somatic exercises lies in their simplicity and flexibility—they can be practiced anytime and anywhere without the need for specialized equipment. It makes somatic exercises a versatile and inclusive tool for fostering well-being and promoting a harmonious connection between the mind and body.

Benefits of Somatic Exercises

As I stated earlier, engaging in somatic exercises offers several benefits for both mental and physical well-being. Here are some key advantages:

1. **Enhanced Body Awareness:** Somatic exercises promote mindfulness and deepen one's awareness of bodily sensations. This heightened awareness allows individuals to better understand and respond to signals from their bodies, fostering a more profound connection between the mind and body.

2. **Stress Reduction:** Somatic exercises often incorporate relaxation techniques to reduce stress levels. Mindful movements and breathwork can help

alleviate tension, calm the nervous system, and promote relaxation and tranquility.

3. **Improved Posture and Flexibility:** Many somatic exercises enhance posture, flexibility, and range of motion. By addressing muscular imbalances and promoting proper alignment, these exercises contribute to improved posture, flexibility, and overall physical mobility.

4. **Pain Management:** Somatics particularly benefit individuals with chronic pain or discomfort. The practice helps identify and release tension held in the muscles, providing relief from pain associated with various conditions, such as muscular tension, headaches, and joint discomfort.

5. **Emotional Regulation:** Somatic exercises can positively impact emotional well-being by encouraging the release of physical and emotional tension stored in the body. It can contribute to emotional regulation, helping individuals manage stress, anxiety, and other emotional challenges more effectively.

6. **Trauma Recovery:** Somatic therapy, a form of somatic exercises, is recognized for its effectiveness in trauma recovery. The gentle and mindful approach allows individuals to process and release trauma held in the body, fostering healing and resilience.

7. **Accessible for All Ages and Fitness Levels:** One of the notable advantages of somatic exercises is their accessibility. These exercises are designed to be inclusive, accommodating individuals of all ages, abilities, and fitness levels. They can be adapted to suit individual needs and preferences.

8. **Increased Mind-Body Connection:** Somatic exercises promote a deeper understanding of the intricate relationship between physical sensations, emotions, and thoughts. This increased mind-body connection contributes to a holistic approach to health and well-being.

9. **Versatility and Convenience:** Somatic exercises do not require specialized equipment, making them convenient to practice anytime, anywhere. This versatility allows individuals to easily incorporate somatic exercises into their daily routines.

Basics of Somatic Movement

Before you begin doing somatic exercises, it's important to understand the basics of somatic movement. Somatic movement isn't about following specific poses or routines; it's about discovering and feeling your body thoughtfully and playfully.

Somatic movement revolves around three main ideas: breathing, grounding, and scanning. In this guide, you'll discover what these principles involve, why they matter, and how to use them in your somatic exercises.

1. Breathing

Breathing is super important for life, and it's a really powerful tool for somatic movement, which is all about understanding and feeling your body. How you breathe can affect how you feel physically, mentally, and emotionally, and it works the other way around. If you change how you breathe, you can change how you feel, think, and move.

Breathing can do different things for you:

1. **Relax and Release Tension:** Breathing deeply and slowly can activate your parasympathetic nervous system, like the body's rest and recovery mode. It can help lower your pulse rate, blood pressure, and stress levels, calming you and relieving muscle and mind tension.

2. **Energize and Invigorate:** Breathing rapidly and forcefully can activate your sympathetic nervous system, like the body's fight or flight mode. It can increase your pulse rate, blood pressure, and alertness, giving you a burst of energy and invigorating your body and mind.

3. **Balance and Harmonize:** Breathing rhythmically and evenly can create a state of coherence where your heart, head, and body are all in sync. It can boost your

mood, thinking, and immunity, helping you balance and harmonize your body and mind.

When practicing breathing in somatic movement, you need to pay attention to four things: how fast you breathe, how deep you breathe, the pattern of your breath, and where you breathe. You can try different combinations of these aspects and see how they affect your body and mind. For instance:

- Breathing steadily and deeply into your abdomen in a regular pattern can help you relax and release tension.

- Breathing rapidly and shallowly into your chest in an irregular pattern can help you energize and invigorate.

- Breathing moderately and thoroughly into your whole body in a balanced pattern can help you balance and harmonize.

You can also sync your breath with your movements:

1. Inhale as you lift your limbs, exhale as you lower them to create a smooth and fluid motion.

2. Exhale as you rotate your torso, inhale as you return to the center to deepen your movement and create a strong and dynamic motion.

3. Inhale as you gather into a bundle, exhale as you expand into a star to add variety and expression to your movement.

2. Grounding

Grounding is all about connecting with the earth or whatever surface you're on. It helps you feel more stable, secure, and supported, making your movements smoother and more effective.

Here's how grounding can be useful:

1. **Stabilize and Support:** Grounding helps create a strong and stable foundation for your movements. It distributes your weight and force, preventing stumbling or injuries and making your movements more comfortable and confident.

2. **Align and Organize:** Grounding allows you to align and organize your body parts in relation to the earth. It improves your posture, balance, and coordination, making your movements more accurate and precise.

3. **Perceive and Respond:** Grounding helps you sense and respond to feedback from the earth. It enhances your awareness, perception, and ability to adapt, making your movements more sensitive and responsive.

To practice grounding in somatic movement, focus on three aspects of your connection with the earth: the quality, the quantity, and the direction. Experiment with different combinations and observe how they affect your body and mind. For instance:

- Gentle and light contact with a small area, pressing away from the earth, creates a delicate and airy movement, giving a sense of lightness and freedom.

- Firm and weighty contact with a large area, drawing towards the earth, creates a strong and grounded movement, offering a sense of heaviness and solidity.

- Medium and moderate contact with a balanced area, gliding along the earth, creates a seamless and fluent movement, providing a sense of neutrality and harmony.

You can also use your contact with the earth to start, go along with, or finish your movements. For example:

1. Push off the earth as you leap, landing gently, creating a forceful and dynamic movement and a sense of enthusiasm and exhilaration.

2. Slide along the earth as you roll, feeling its texture and temperature, creating a lively and exploratory movement and a sense of inquiry and discovery.

3. Rest on the earth as you lie down, feeling its support and solace, creating a relaxing and calming movement and a sense of serenity and harmony.

3. Scanning

Scanning means looking closely at and checking out your body, both inside and out. It helps you understand yourself better and take care of yourself. Scanning can also make your movements better and more varied.

Here's how scanning can help you:

1. **Observe and Examine:** Scanning helps you look at and explore different body parts—how they look, feel, and work. It helps you recognize your strengths, limits, preferences, and needs. It lets you adjust your movements to make them better and more effective.

2. **Release and Relax:** Scanning can ease your body's tension, pain, or discomfort. It helps restore your energy and vitality, preventing and healing injuries. It improves your overall health and well-being.

3. **Explore and Experiment:** Scanning allows you to try different ways of moving your body. You discover new possibilities and potentials, challenging and overcoming your limits and fears. It boosts your creativity and expression.

To do scanning in somatic movement, focus on two things: where you're looking and how you're looking. Try different combinations and see how they affect your body and mind. For instance:

- **Focusing on a Specific Body Part:** Look at, say, your hand and move it in different directions—up, down, left, right, forward, backward. This creates a detailed and precise movement, making you feel clear and focused.

- **Focusing on Your Whole Body:** Look at your entire body and move it in one direction, like forward. This creates a general and overall movement, making you feel simple and unified.

- **Focusing on Various Body Parts:** Look at different body parts and move them in different directions. For example, move your head left, your torso right, your limbs up, and your legs down. This creates a complex and varied movement, making you feel diverse.

You can also use your looking and exploring to start, go along with, or finish your movements. For example:

- **Looking at Your Hand:** Follow your hand's movement with your eyes. It creates a curious and attentive movement, making you feel interested and engaged.

- **Feeling Your Spine:** Sense your spine's movement with your awareness. It creates a subtle and refined movement, making you feel subtle and refined.

Imagining Your Heart: Picture your heart's movement with your imagination. It creates an expressive and emotional movement, making you feel expressive and emotional.

CHAPTER 2: DIFFERENT SOMATIC EXERCISES

Neck Release

The neck release exercise is also known as letting go of tension in your neck. It is like giving stress a break, boosting your energy, and making you feel more relaxed. This exercise is all about easing tension in your neck. It helps stretch your neck, making it more flexible and improving your standing or sitting. It's especially helpful if you spend a lot of time on laptops or smartphones, as it helps undo the strain from keeping your neck in an awkward position.

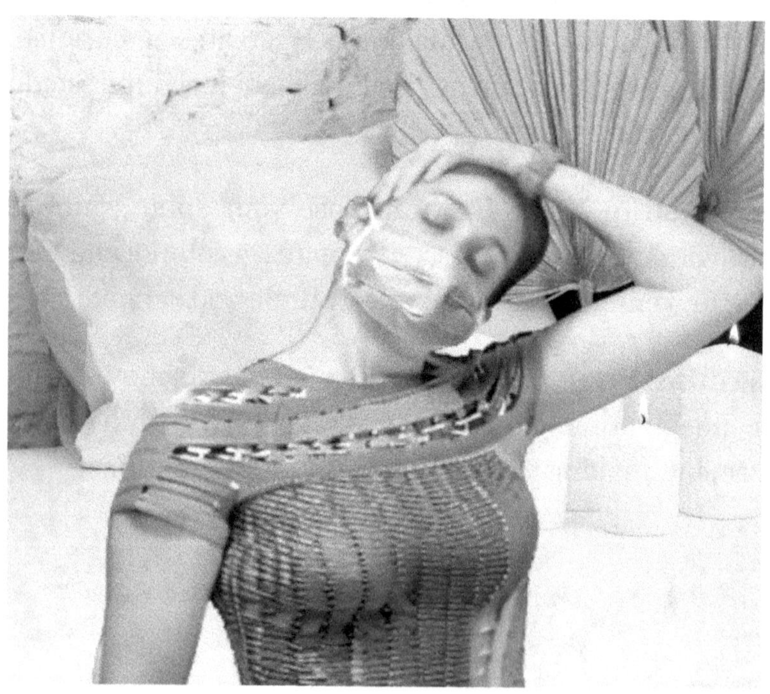

Here are the steps for this exercise:

1. Get comfy sitting or standing, keeping your back straight and shoulders relaxed. Put your right hand on the left side of your head and gently tilt your head to the right. You should feel a gentle stretch on the left side of your neck.

2. When you breathe in, squeeze the left side of your neck against your hand. As you breathe out, relax that squeeze and let your head move more to the right. You'll feel a deeper stretch on the left side of your neck.

3. Do this for 3 to 5 breaths or however long feels good. Then, switch sides and do the same on your right side.

Back Arch

The back arch, a simple yet effective exercise, involves lying on your back, bending your knees, and lifting your lower back off the ground, creating a gentle arch. This movement offers various benefits for the body. It helps alleviate tension in the lower back and abdomen, relieving discomfort. The back arch also improves flexibility in the lower back and pelvis, promoting better posture and alignment.

Here are the steps to practice this exercise:

1. Lie on your back with your knees bent and your heels flat on the ground. Put your arms beside you and relax your

shoulders. Ensure your back is flat and your head is aligned with your spine.

2. Breathe in and push your lower back into the floor while tilting your pelvis towards your head. You should feel a gentle stretch in your lower back and stomach.

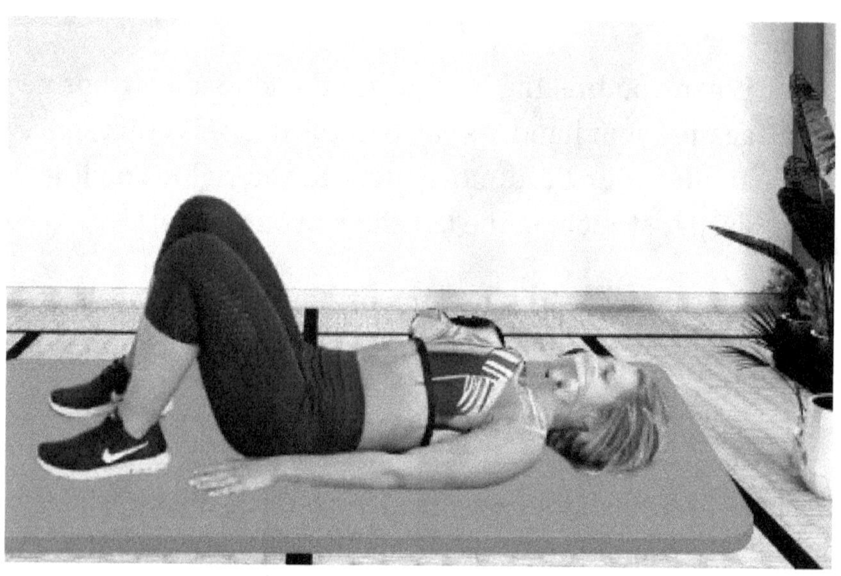

3. Breathe out and lift your lower back off the floor, turning your pelvis away from your head. You'll feel a gentle stretch in your lower back and pelvis.

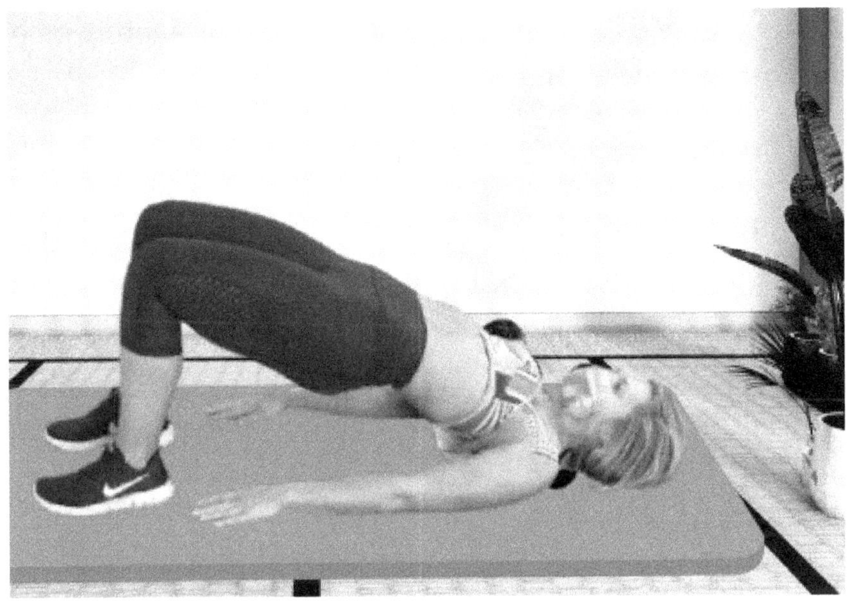

4. Do this for 10 to 20 breaths or as long as it feels good. Notice how your lower back and pelvis feel, and see how your breath goes along with your movement.

Hamstring Stretch

The hamstring stretch is a beneficial exercise involving the elongation of the muscles at the back of the thigh. This stretch is typically performed by sitting on the floor and reaching towards the toes. It enhances the flexibility of the hamstrings, promoting a wider range of motion in the legs.

This increased flexibility contributes to better posture and alignment, reducing the risk of strain or injury. Regular practice of hamstring stretches can alleviate muscle tension, particularly in the lower back, and enhance overall leg mobility.

Moreover, it aids in preventing stiffness and promoting blood circulation in the leg muscles.

Here are the steps for this exercise:

1. Lie on your back with your legs straight out in front of you and your arms at your sides.

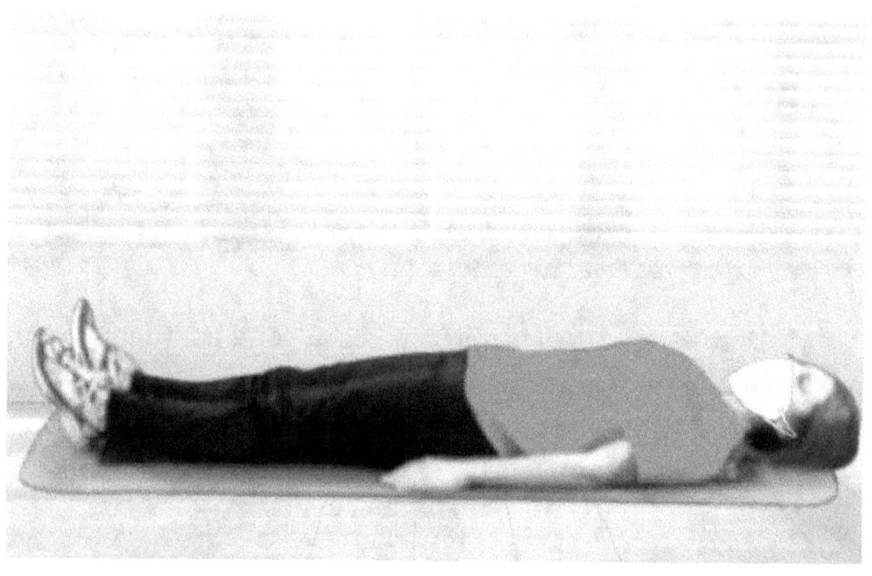

2. Slowly raise one leg as high as is comfortable while keeping the other leg on the floor. Use your hands to support the raised leg, placing them around the thigh or calf. Gently stretch by pulling with your hands, feeling a slight pull in the back of your thigh. Continue to breathe steadily while in this position, ensuring your knee remains as straight as possible without locking it. Hold the stretch, slowly counting to 5.

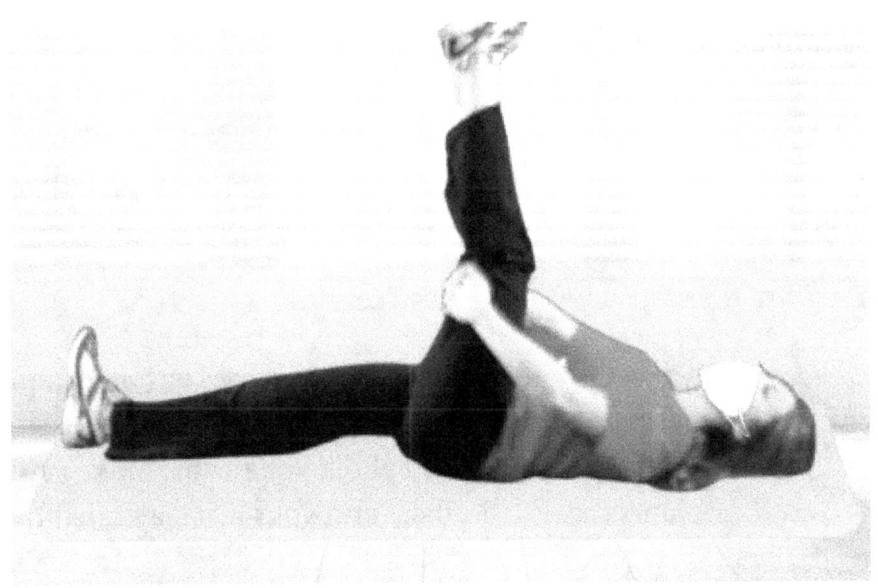

3. Release the stretch with control. Return the leg to the floor and repeat the sequence 5 times on each side. If reaching around your leg is challenging, use a towel. Wrap it around your leg and pull it against the towel to achieve the stretch.

Chest Opener

The Chest Opener is a beneficial exercise designed to stretch and open up the chest muscles, typically performed by interlacing the fingers behind the back and lifting the arms slightly. This simple yet effective stretch comes with several advantages for the body. It promotes improved posture by counteracting the forward-leaning position often associated with activities like prolonged sitting or desk work.

By expanding the chest, the stretch helps relieve tension in the shoulders and upper back, reducing the risk of stiffness and discomfort. Additionally, the Chest Opener enhances respiratory function by allowing deeper breaths and expanding lung capacity.

Here are the steps to practice this exercise:

1. Stand or sit comfortably with your back straight and shoulders relaxed. Put your hands behind your back, fingers interlaced, and straighten your arms. Make sure your palms face each other, and your arms are slightly bent.

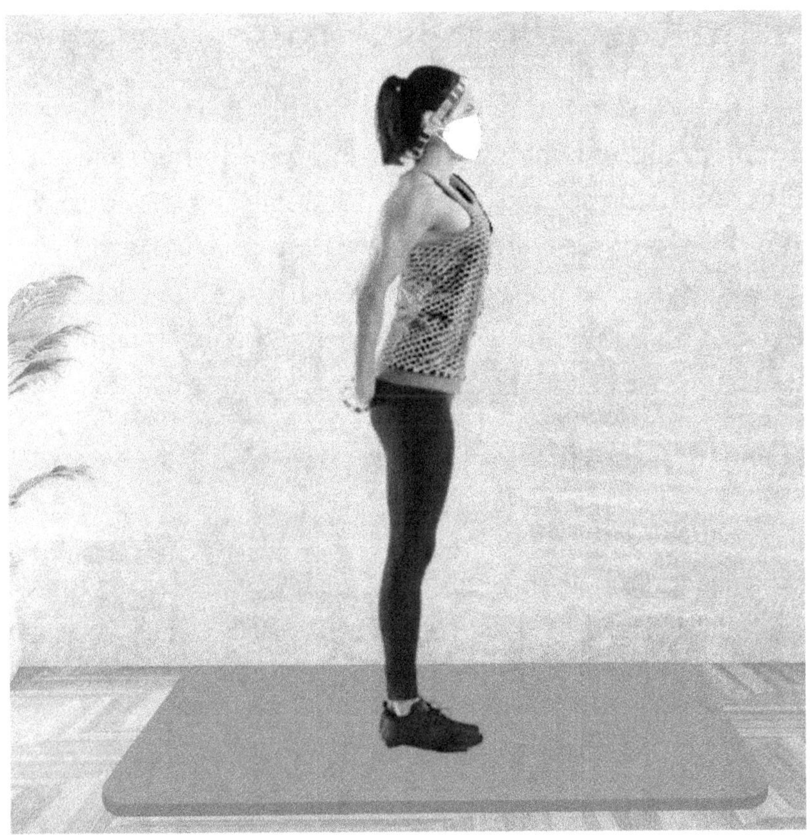

2. Breathe in and squeeze your chest, shoulders, and arms, bringing your palms towards your hips. You'll feel a gentle stretch in your chest, shoulders, and arms.

3. Breathe out, lift your palms away from your hips, and pull your shoulder blades together. You'll feel a gentle stretch in your chest, shoulders, and arms.

4. Do this for 10 to 20 breaths or as long as it feels good. Notice how your chest, shoulders, and arms feel and how your breathing accompanies your movement.

Hip Flexor Stretch

The Hip Flexor Stretch is a valuable exercise aimed at stretching and enhancing the flexibility of the muscles at the hip's front. This stretch involves kneeling on one knee while extending the opposite leg behind, allowing for a controlled and gentle stretch. The stretch contributes to improved posture and reduced strain on the lower back, supporting overall spinal health.

Here are the steps for practicing this exercise:

1. Kneel on the floor with your right leg bent and your left leg stretched out behind you. Put your hands on your right thigh and lean a bit forward. Keep your back straight and your head in line with your spine.

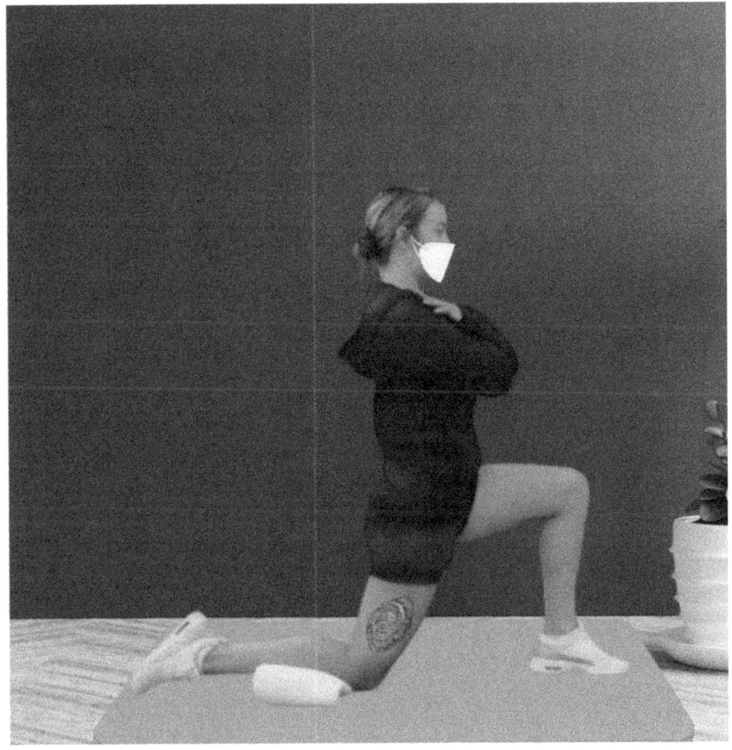

2. Breathe in, tighten your left hip, thigh, and groin muscles, and press your left leg into the floor. You'll feel a gentle stretch in your left hip, thigh, and groin.

3. Breathe out, relax those muscles, and let your pelvis move forward. You'll feel a deeper stretch in your left hip, thigh, and groin.

4. Do this for 3 to 5 breaths or as long as it feels good. Then, switch sides and do the same for your right hip, thigh, and groin.

Baby Stretch

The baby stretch is a wonderful exercise for stretching and releasing tension in your body. It's a simple yet effective way to alleviate tightness caused by stress and trauma. As we go through challenging experiences, our muscles tend to tighten up, and this exercise helps release those negative emotions, leaving you feeling more energized.

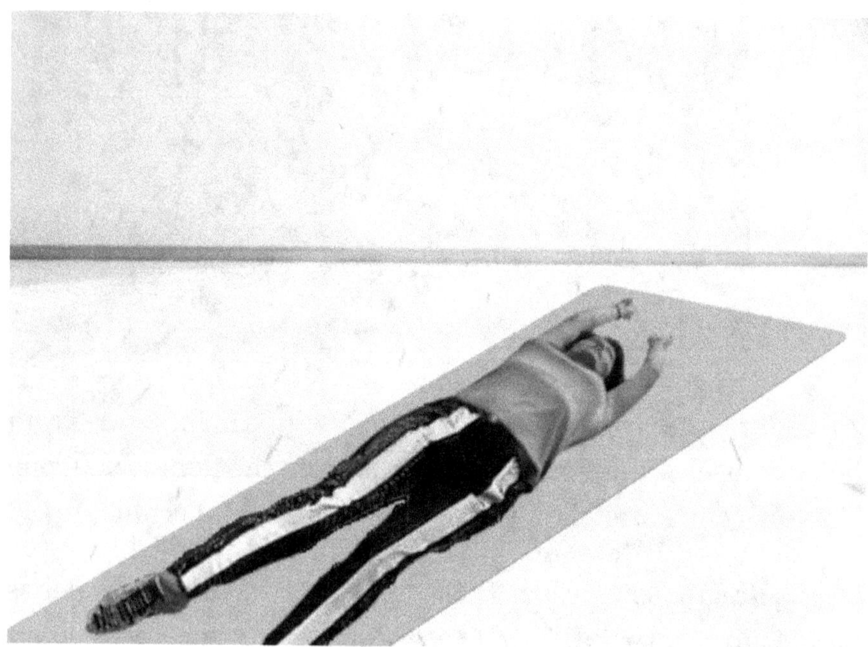

This stretch is so natural that even babies instinctively do it. It indicates that you might benefit even more if it doesn't feel comfortable initially. Along with emotional release, the baby stretch improves your posture and aligns your body, contributing to overall well-being.

Here are the steps to practice this exercise:

1. Begin by lying on your back with your legs spread wider than shoulder-width apart. Keep your arms straight and resting next to your body.

2. Reach over your head and stretch your arms, legs, and feet simultaneously, as if you're reaching for something just out of grasp. Imagine the complete stretch experienced by a baby after waking up. Hold this stretched position for about 5 seconds, allowing your body to fully extend.

3. Return to the starting position, releasing the stretch. Repeat the exercise for the recommended number of times, focusing on gently releasing any tension or tightness during each stretch. Emulate the natural and comfortable movements akin to a baby waking up and stretching.

Pelvic Preparation

Pelvic preparation is an excellent exercise to enhance your connection with the pelvis and lower back. The main goal is to bring attention to your breath uniquely. The exercise encourages mindful breathing by inhaling during arching and exhaling as you relax.

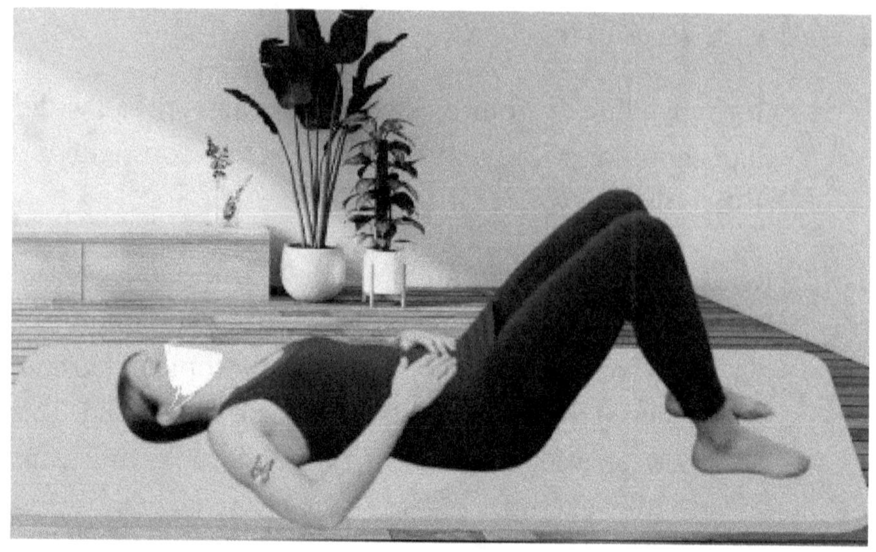

Here are the steps for practicing this exercise:

1. Begin by lying on your back with your legs bent, and ensure your feet are fully grounded on the floor. After the demonstration, place your left hand at the bottom of your chest and your right hand on your pelvis.

2. Squeeze your pelvic muscles toward the floor while exhaling fully through your mouth. This action helps engage your core and release tension. Maintain this position for approximately 5 seconds.

3. Release the tension in your core, and inhale deeply through your nose. Allow your body to relax while focusing on your breath. Hold this position for about 5 seconds.

4. Perform the pelvic squeeze, exhale, and subsequent release for the recommended repetitions. Pay attention to the rhythm of your breath and the subtle movements in your pelvic region. Consistent practice of this pelvic preparation exercise can contribute to improved core strength, enhanced breath awareness, and a release of tension in the pelvic area.

Moving Rock

The moving rock exercise is designed to enhance your balance and flexibility, while also engaging your core muscles. It offers specific benefits for your lower back by releasing tension and stress, making it particularly helpful for preventing and relieving lower back pain.

Here's how to do it:

1. Lie on your back on a comfortable mat. Bring your knees toward your chest, keeping your feet flat on the mat. Ensure your spine is in contact with the mat throughout the exercise.

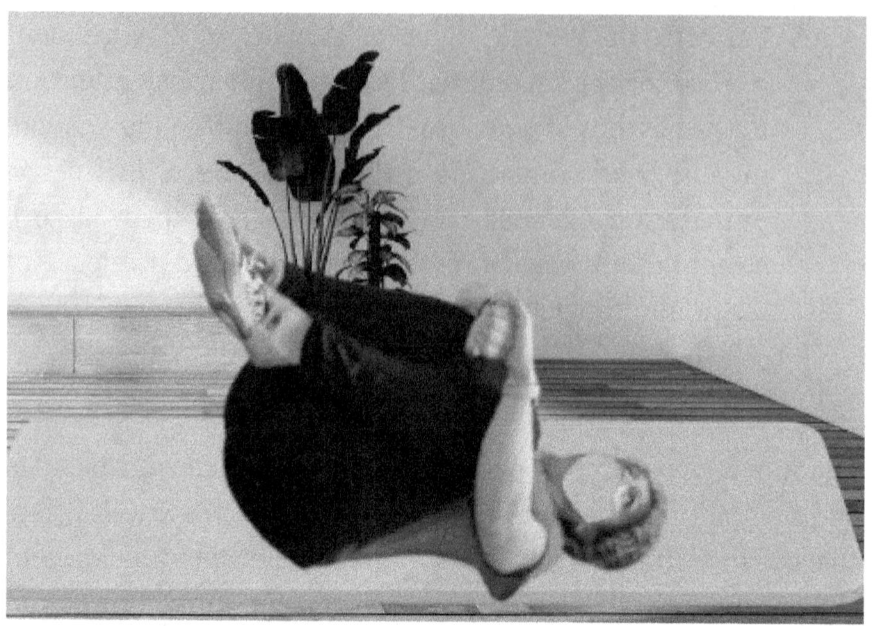

2. Gently start rocking your body from side to side. The movement should be smooth and controlled, creating a rocking motion while keeping your balance. Throughout the exercise, focus on maintaining balance. The rocking motion should feel good and easy, promoting relaxation.

3. Continue rocking from side to side, alternating the movement to each side. It helps engage different muscles and promotes a balanced workout.

4. Move gently and slowly to maximize the effectiveness of the exercise. Avoid sudden or jerky movements, allowing your muscles to work in a controlled manner.

5. Repeat the rocking motion for the specified duration or number of repetitions. Consistency is key, so aim for a steady and controlled pace throughout the exercise.

Despair

Despair, often linked to distress and discouragement, can be effectively addressed through a simple exercise that promotes letting go. These emotions, when not dealt with, tend to manifest in the neck, leading to stress and pain. By releasing these negative feelings through the suggested exercise, one addresses emotional well-being and experiences physical benefits.

Here's how to do this exercise:

1. Begin by finding a quiet and comfortable space to perform the despair exercise. Place a mat on the floor and sit with your legs crossed, ensuring your back is upright.

2. Position both hands on the back of your head, with your elbows pointing outward. Gently drop your head forward until your chin touches your collarbone. Allow your neck muscles to relax in this position, finding a comfortable and natural stretch.

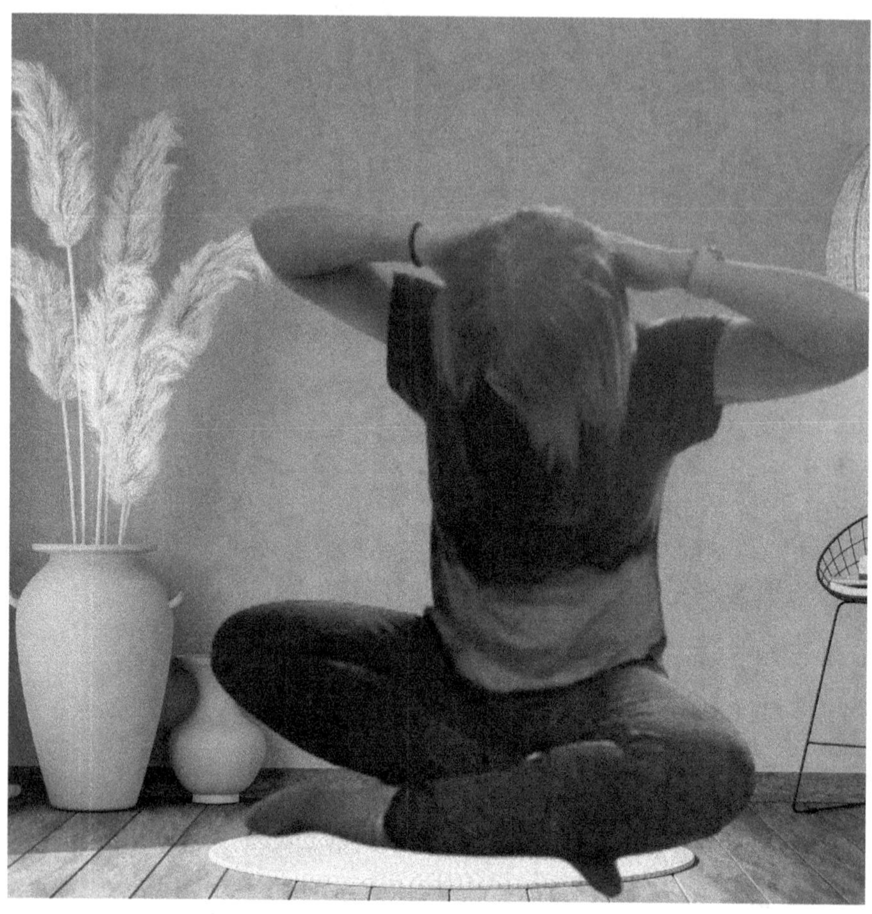

3. Inhale slowly and, while maintaining the hand placement on the back of your head, turn your face to the left. As you do this, you will feel a gentle stretch on the sides of your neck. Hold this position for a few breaths, allowing the stretch to deepen.

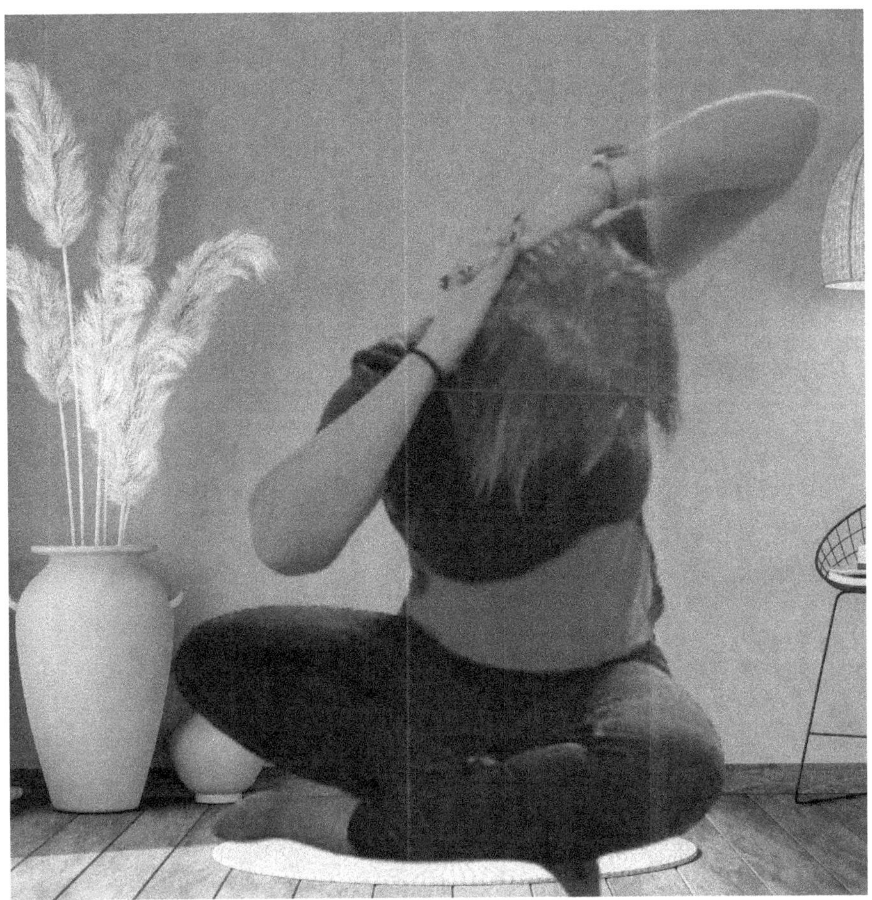

4. Exhale gradually as you return to the starting position with your head upright. Ensure that the movement is slow and controlled to maximize the benefits of the exercise.

5. Repeat the exercise by turning your face to the right while inhaling. Feel the stretch on the opposite side of your neck. Exhale as you return to the starting position.

Superman

The Superman exercise is a fantastic workout that benefits your body. Lifting your chest, arms, and legs off the ground simultaneously strengthens your upper back, glutes, and hamstrings. It improves your posture and targets muscles that are sometimes overlooked.

Here are the steps to practice this exercise:

1. Begin by lying on your belly with your legs extended. Place your cheek on the mat and position your hand facing down on the mat.

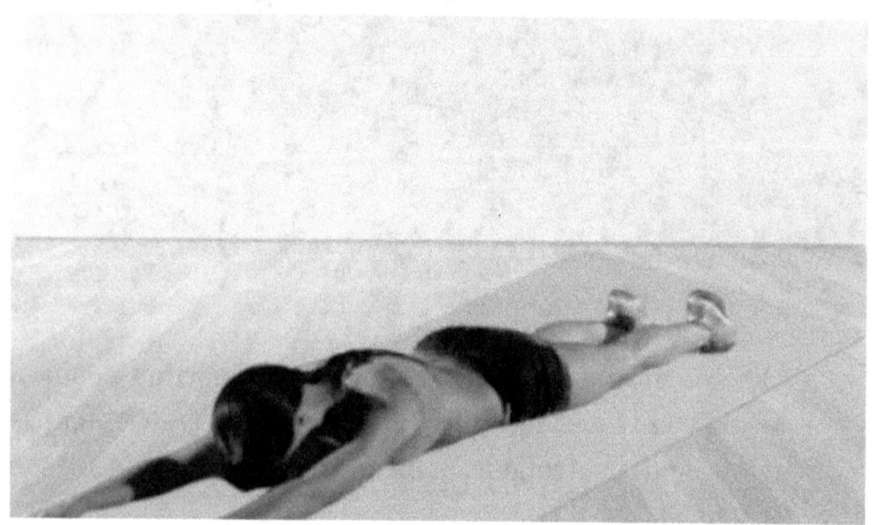

2. Llift your neck and your arm simultaneously. Allow your hand to touch your cheek while raising your leg straight off the mat. Maintain this position for 3 to 5 seconds, engaging your core muscles for stability.

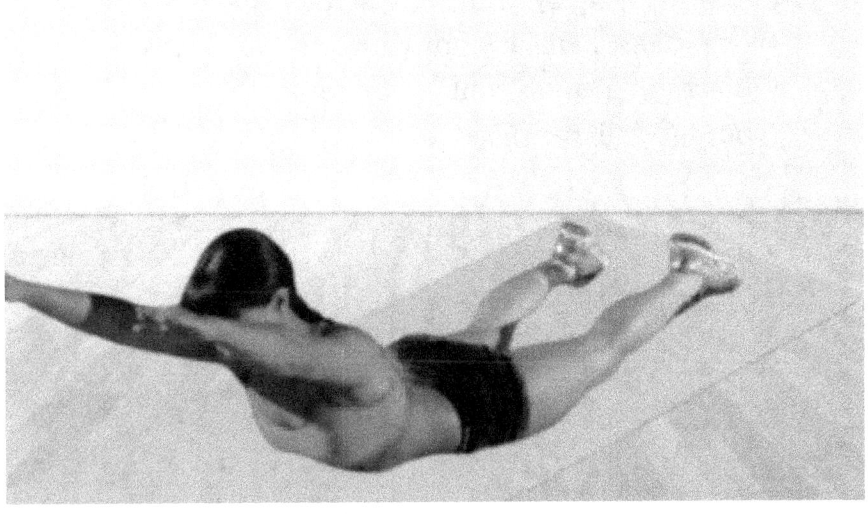

3. Repeat the exercise for the specified number of repetitions, gradually increasing as your strength improves. Focus on maintaining proper form and control throughout each repetition.

4. Repeat the exercise on the other side to work both sides of your body evenly.

Side Reach

Side reach is a simple, fluid exercise emphasizing smooth motion and is not commonly used in everyday activities. Unlike some exercises, it doesn't demand a specific level of strength or flexibility, making it accessible for most people. The key is to keep the body relaxed and maintain controlled breathing without tensing up during the movement.

Here's how you can do it:

1. Begin by lying on your right side in a fetal position with your knees bent at approximately 90 degrees. Extend your right arm in front of you for support. Fully stretch your left arm overhead.

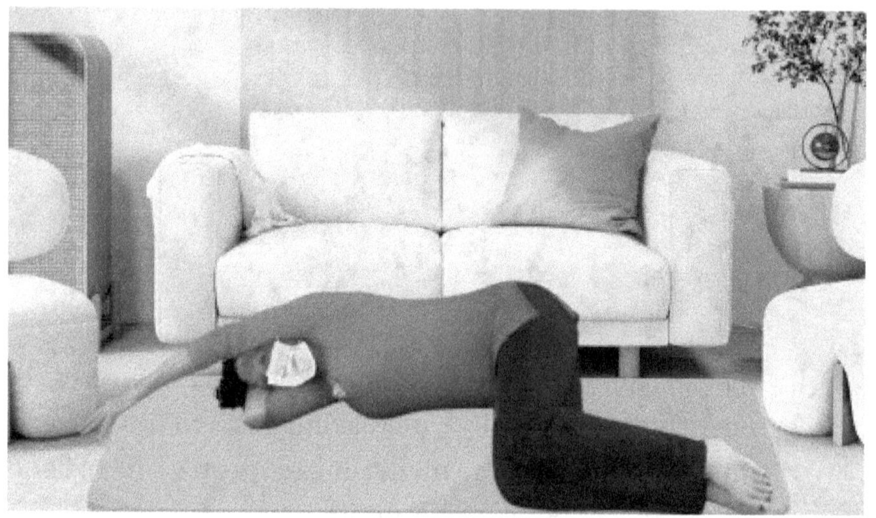

2. Lift your head to stretch the right side of your neck while raising your left ankle as much as possible. Reach towards your left ankle with your left hand, keeping your knees together throughout the movement.

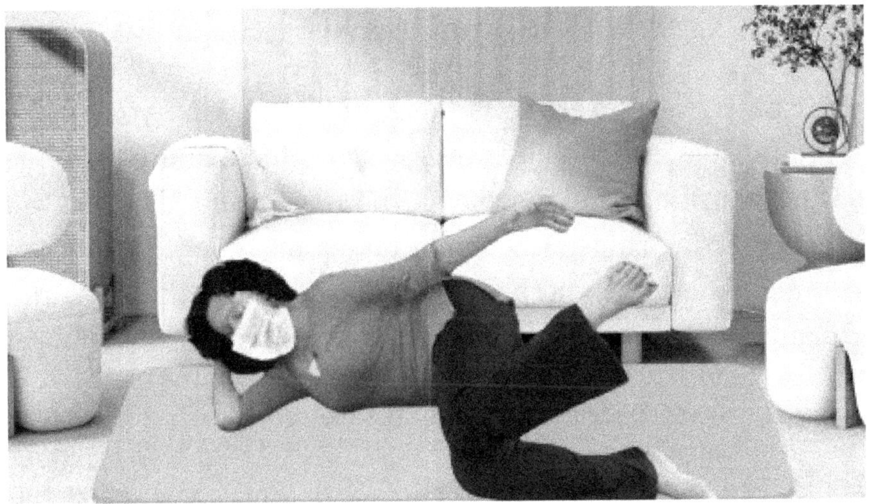

3. Slowly return to the starting position after touching your left ankle with your left hand. Perform the lifting and reaching movement for the specified number of repetitions, focusing on controlled and deliberate motions. It engages the muscles along your side and enhances flexibility.

4. To ensure balanced development, transition to your left side and repeat the exercise. Begin in a fetal position with your knees bent, extend your left arm for support, and fully stretch your right arm overhead. Lift your head, raise your right ankle, and reach towards it with your right hand. Return to the starting position and repeat as directed.

Spinal Wave

The spinal wave exercise is fantastic for making your spine more flexible and mobile, preventing stiffness and pain while easing tension. The movement becomes smoother as you practice, though mastering it may take some time. This exercise is one of the top choices for maintaining a healthy back and enhancing your overall connection with your body.

Here are the steps for practicing this exercise:

1. Begin in a standing position with your arms relaxed at the sides of your body. Ensure your entire body is straight, from your head down to your feet.

2. Move your upper chest forward in a gentle, flowing motion. Allow this movement to create a wave-like effect that travels down your spine. As your upper chest returns to the starting position, simultaneously move your belly forward, creating a continuous and seamless wave-like motion along your spine.

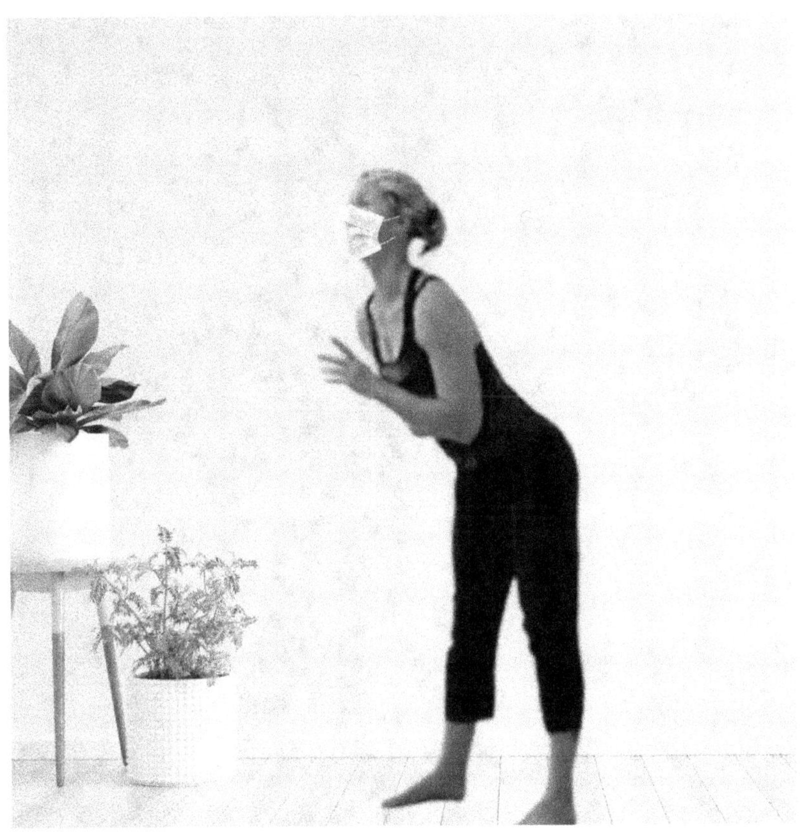

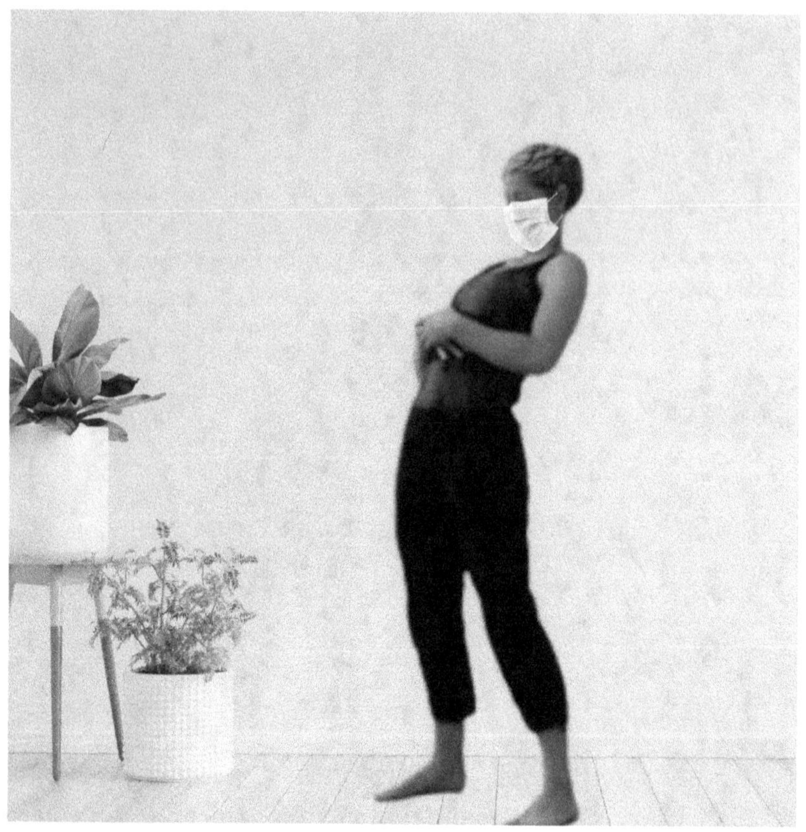

3. The somatic spinal wave exercise is characterized by its fluidity. As you move your upper chest and belly in a coordinated manner, strive for a smooth and uninterrupted wave motion. This fluidity contributes to the flexibility and mobility of your spine.

4. Continue the somatic spinal wave movement for the specified duration, ensuring a controlled and deliberate pace. The repetition of this exercise contributes to improved spinal flexibility, posture, and overall well-being.

Reach Back

The reach-back exercise enhances the flexibility and mobility of your upper back, shoulders, and lower back. To perform it, keep your entire body relaxed and maintain the position of your legs while twisting your back, head, and arms.

Here are the steps to practice this exercise:

1. Begin by sitting on a comfortable mat with your legs extended straight before you. Ensure that your back is straight and your posture is upright.

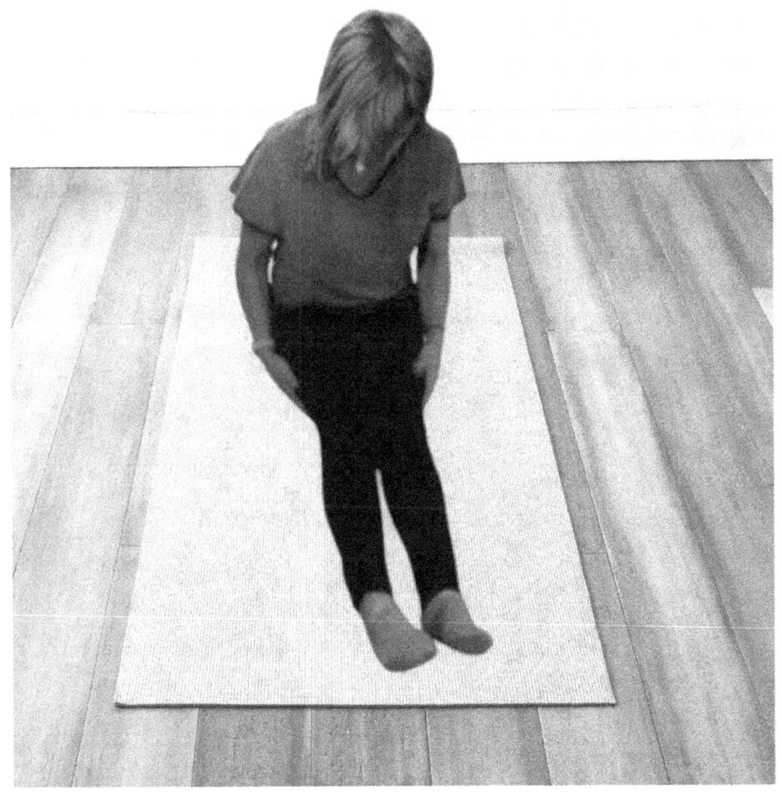

2. Gently twist your torso to the right side while maintaining the straight position of your legs. Place your right hand on the mat beside you for support. This twist engages your core and prepares your spine for the reach-back movement.

3. With your right hand supporting, extend your left hand backward, reaching toward the space behind you. Feel the stretch along your spine and the rotation in your upper body. Keep your movements controlled and within a comfortable range to avoid strain.

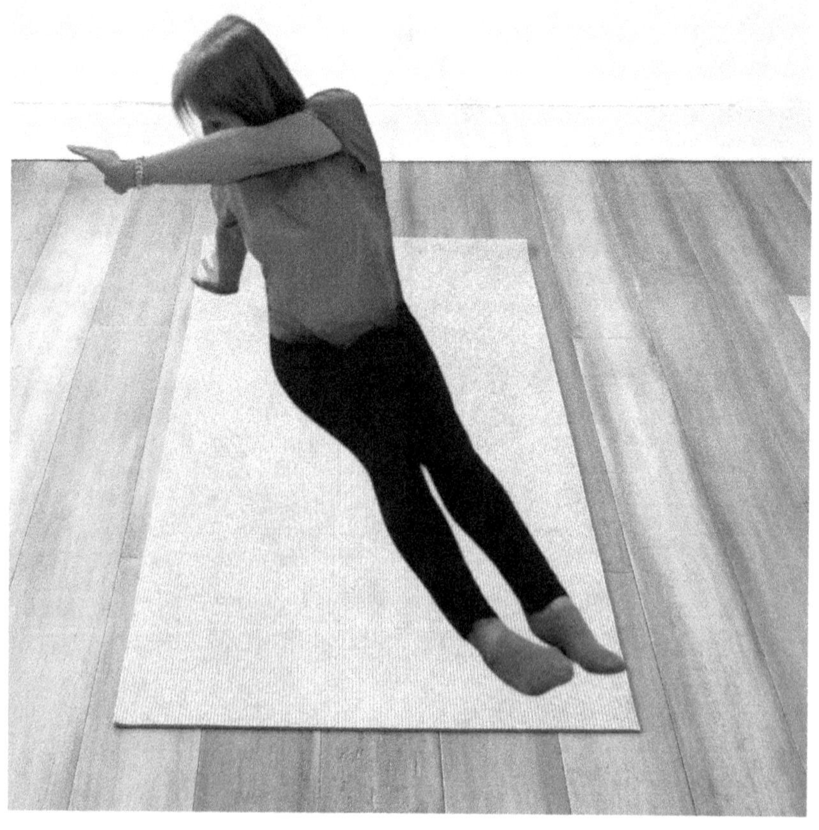

4. Carefully return to the starting position with both hands resting on the mat and your spine in a neutral position. Take a moment to feel the effects of the stretch before proceeding to the other side.

5. Now, twist your torso to the left side while keeping your legs straight. Place your left hand on the mat for support and reach backward with your right hand. Experience the stretch along the opposite side of your spine.

6. Continue alternating between left and right twists, reaching back with the opposite hand each time. Aim for a smooth and controlled motion, focusing on the sensation of the stretch in your spine. Repeat the exercise for a desired number of repetitions, considering your comfort and flexibility.

Standing Reach

The standing reach exercise is designed to boost the flexibility and mobility of your upper body while improving the overall connection and balance with your body. To maximize its benefits, perform the movements slowly and focus on controlled breathing. It's crucial to avoid tensing your neck during the exercise; instead, consciously relax your neck muscles.

Here are the steps for carrying out this exercise:

1. Begin by standing up straight with your feet shoulder-width apart and your hands naturally resting along your body.

2. Raise both arms overhead, keeping them straight. While maintaining straight legs and both feet firmly on the floor, gently bend your torso towards the left side. Allow your left hand to slide down your left leg while reaching with your right hand overhead.

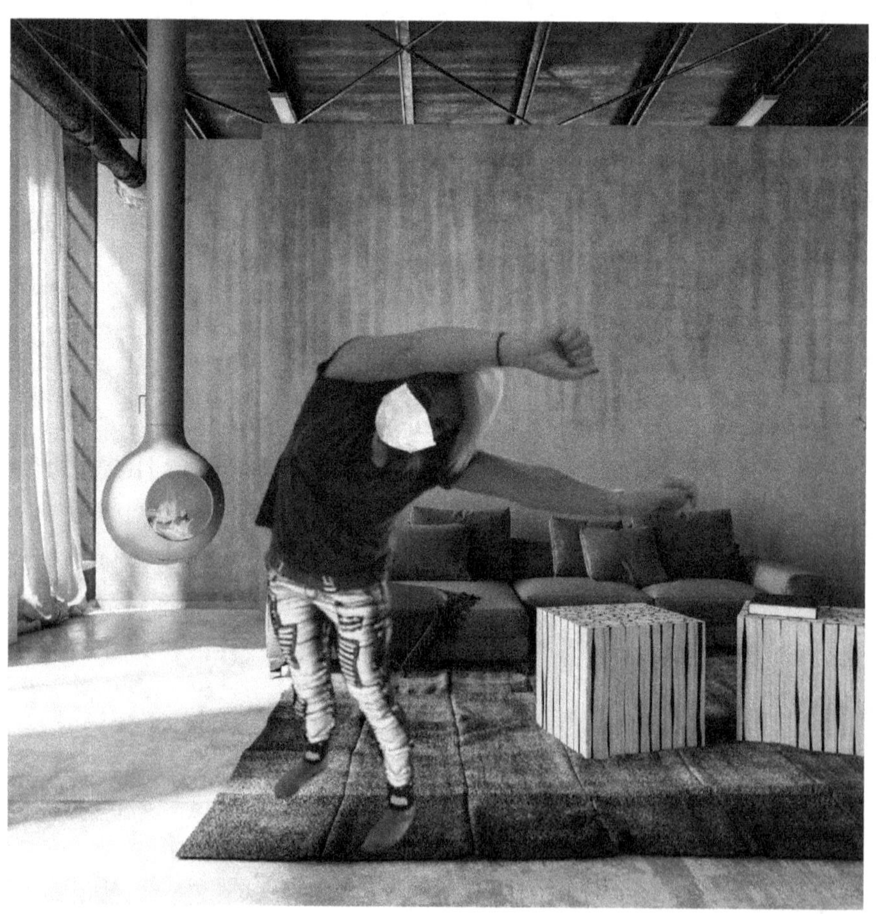

3. Transition smoothly by moving your hands and torso before you, creating a semicircular motion. Visualize drawing a semicircle with your hands as you continue to reach forward.

4. Continue the semicircular motion slowly until you reach the right side. Keep your legs straight, and feel the stretch along your right side.

5. Slowly reverse the movement by creating the semicircle in the opposite direction. Extend your arms overhead and bend to the right, then move your hands and torso across the front until you reach the left side.

6. Continue for the recommended number of repetitions.

Spider Circle

The spider circle exercise is an excellent way to enhance the flexibility and mobility of your upper body, providing relief from tension. It specifically targets the flexibility of your glutes and lower back. It's crucial to avoid tensing your neck during the exercise; instead, consciously relax your neck muscles.

Here are the steps to practice this exercise:

1. Sit comfortably on the mat, cross your legs, and lean your body forward. Reach towards the floor in front of you, gently folding your torso.

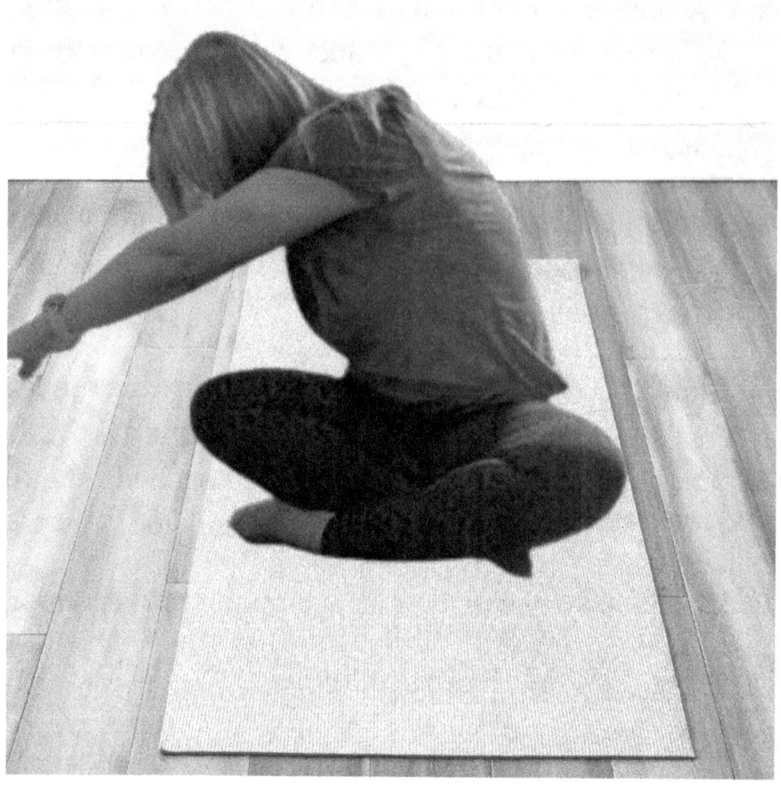

2. Make a smooth movement by rotating your back clockwise, completing a full 360-degree rotation. Use your hands for support as you reach as far as possible, finding a balance between rotation and stability. Feel the stretch and engagement in your torso as you complete the circular motion.

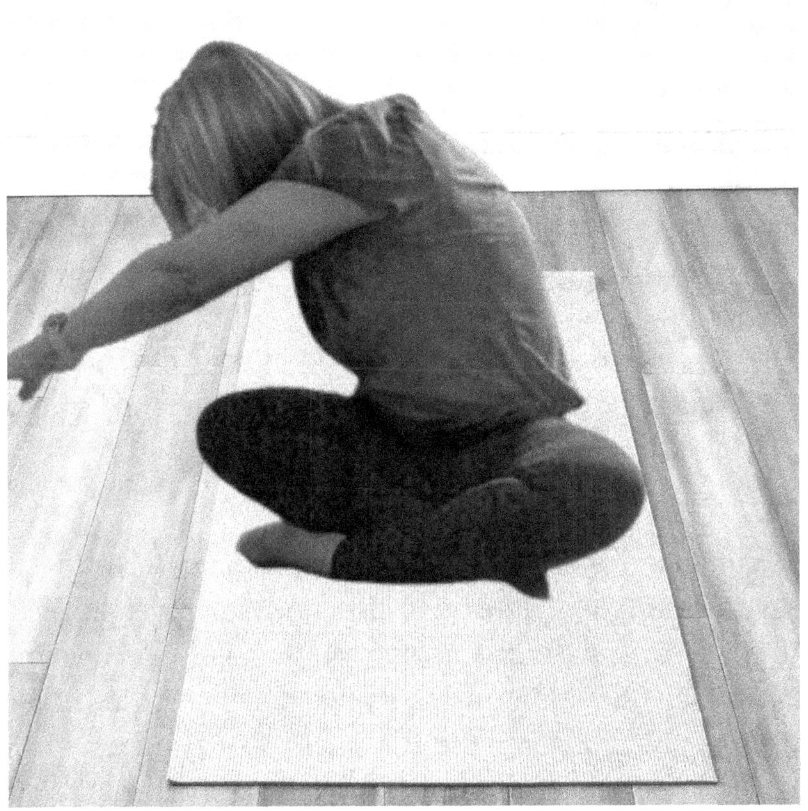

3. While rotating, extend your hands as far as possible without compromising your balance. Once you have completed a full 360-degree clockwise rotation, that counts as one repetition. Take a moment to feel the stretch in your back and sides.

4. Continue the Spider Circle exercise for the specified number of repetitions in a clockwise direction. Keep the motion smooth and controlled, paying attention to the stretch in your back and the engagement of your core.

5. Switch to the counterclockwise direction after completing the specified number of clockwise rotations. Repeat the fluid movement, rotating your back 360 degrees counterclockwise while reaching with your hands.

6. Continue alternating between clockwise and counterclockwise rotations for the specified number of repetitions or as recommended in your fitness routine. Adjust the pace according to your comfort and flexibility.

Star Glute Bridge

The glute bridge is an effective exercise for targeting and strengthening your glutes and groins. Remember to engage your core to maintain the correct position for maximum benefit. Deep breathing helps release tension, so inhale and exhale deeply throughout the movement. Keep your upper body and neck relaxed to optimize the exercise. Adding the glute bridge to your routine can build strength in important muscle groups and improve stability and balance in your lower body.

Here are the steps to practice this exercise:

1. Lie on your back with your legs bent and feet close to each other, fully grounded on the floor. Extend your arms to the sides, creating a 90-degree angle with your body.

2. Inhale deeply and allow your knees to drop sideways, bringing the soles of your feet together. Feel the stretch

in your groin area, and don't worry if your lower back has a slight arch. Hold this position for 2 seconds, maintaining steady and soft breathing.

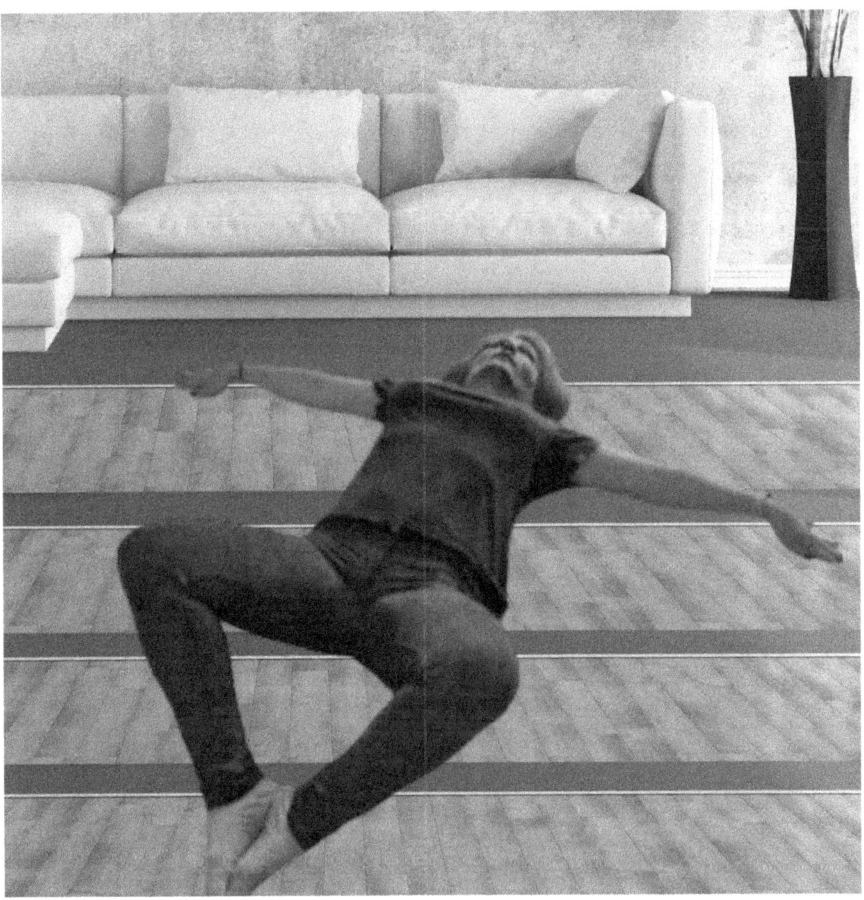

3. Inhale again and lift your hips off the ground while keeping the soles of your feet together and knees open. Ensure that your arms remain in the same extended position on the sides. Feel the contraction in your glutes as you raise your hips.

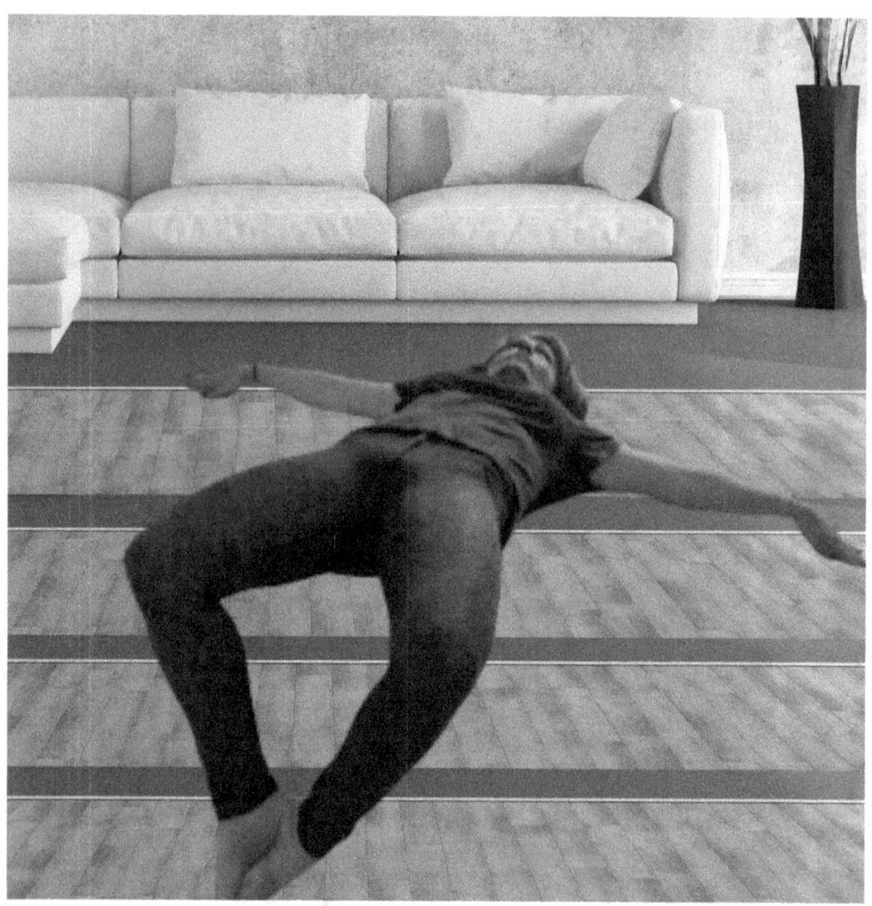

4. Exhale fully and slowly lower your buttocks back to the mat. Control the movement as you return your knees to the starting position. Pay attention to the controlled descent, engaging your muscles throughout.

5. Now, you've completed one repetition! Repeat the sequence for the recommended number of times, maintaining the slow and controlled pace.

Standing Stress Release

The standing stress release exercise is all about letting go of optimal benefits. Start by emptying your mind and consciously relaxing your entire body, focusing on the upper body. As you perform the exercise, imagine shaking off any negative feelings you may carry by incorporating twists and turns into the movements.

Here are the steps for practicing this exercise:

1. Begin in a standing position with your feet slightly wider than shoulder-width apart. Ensure a stable base in your lower body while keeping your weight evenly distributed between both feet.

2. Allow your back and upper body to gently collapse and fall downward. Let your arms relax and hang naturally towards the ground, fully releasing tension in your shoulders and neck. Keep your lower body engaged to maintain balance while intentionally relaxing your upper body and head.

3. Find a comfortable position where your upper body feels relaxed. Hold this position for 5-10 seconds, focusing on releasing tension and letting go of any muscle stress. Breathe naturally and allow your body to relax during this time fully.

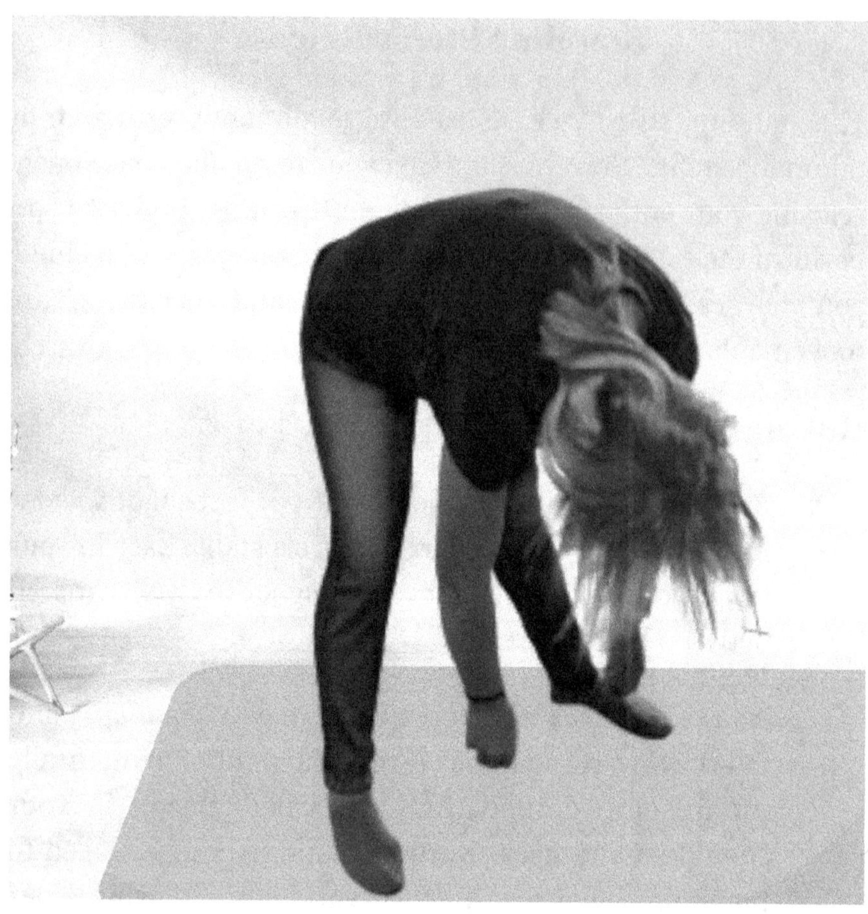

4. While maintaining the collapsed position, twist and turn your upper body towards one side. Hold the twisted position for 2 seconds, feeling a gentle stretch in your torso. Slowly rotate towards the other side, holding for 2 seconds again.

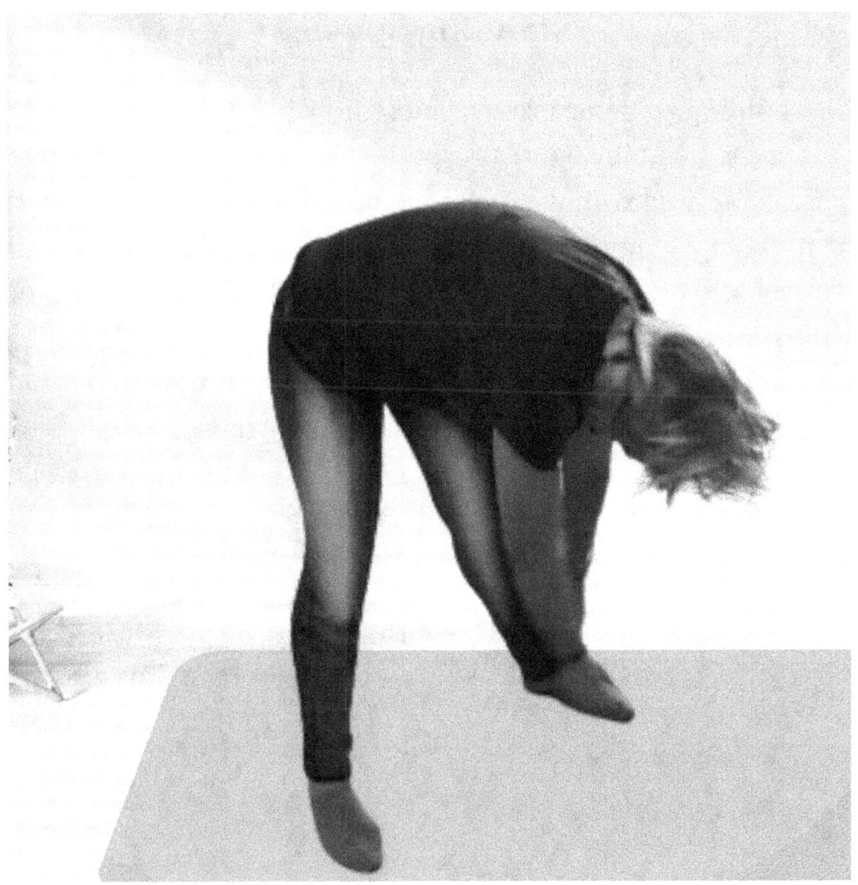

5. Gradually come back to the starting position, returning to a standing stance. Ensure a smooth and controlled movement as you return to the initial standing posture.

6. Repeat the entire sequence for the recommended number of repetitions. Focus on the rhythm of your breath and the intentional release of stress with each repetition.

Standing Spider

The standing spider exercise is incredibly helpful for improving hamstring flexibility and preserving knee health. It involves controlled micro-movements while holding a stretched position, challenging your balance. It's important to keep your neck relaxed and maintain strong ankles with heels on the floor while doing this exercise. In addition to the physical benefits, the standing spider exercise can also release stored anger and negative emotions in the posterior chain of your body.

Here are the steps to practice this exercise:

1. Begin from a standing position with your feet slightly wider than shoulder-width apart. Keep your knees straight as possible while placing both palms on the floor.

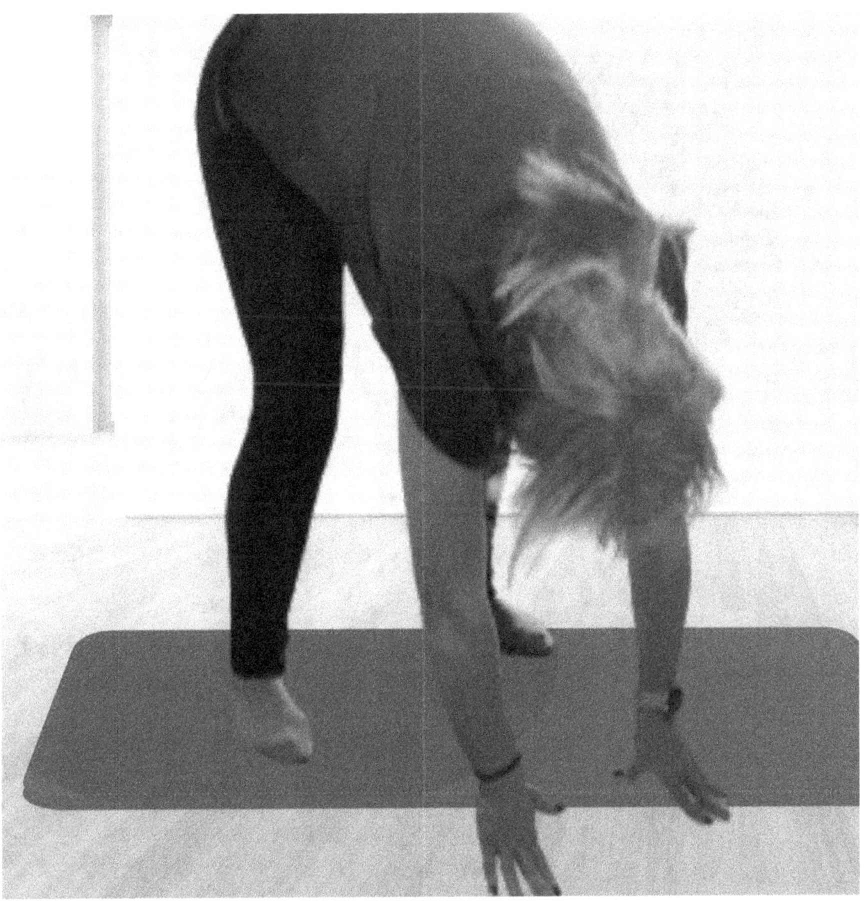

2. From the starting position, slightly bend one knee while maintaining the other knee straight. This movement creates a dynamic stretch in the back of the straight leg and engages the bent leg.

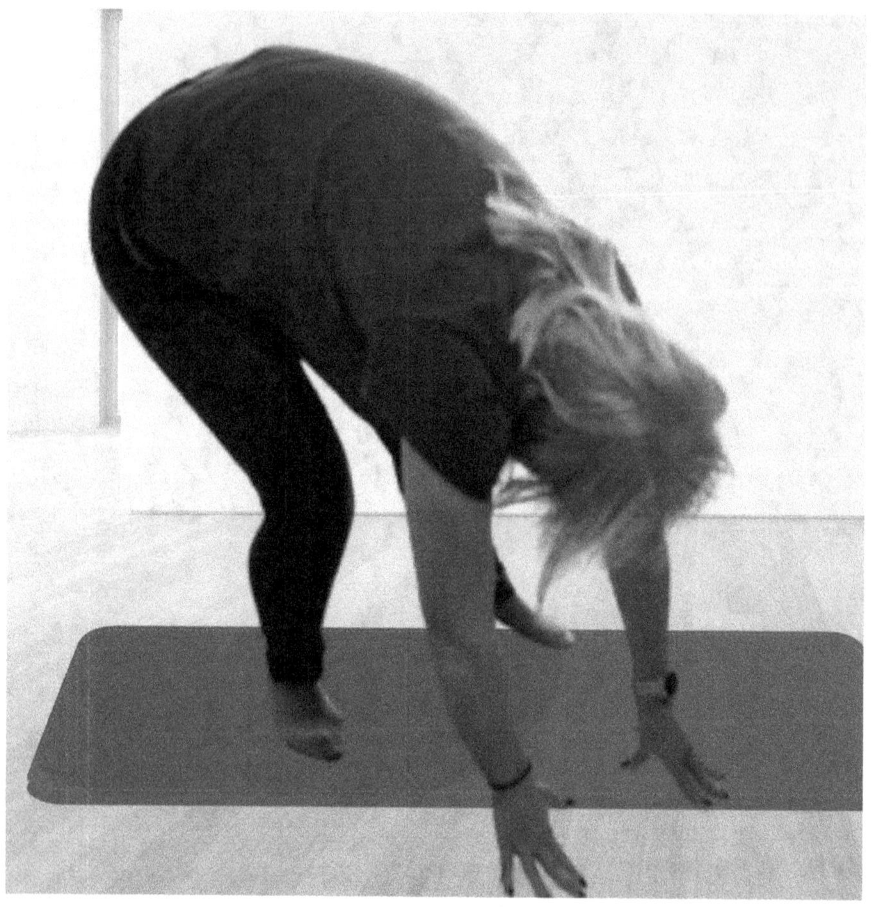

3. After bending one knee, return it to the straight position while simultaneously bending the other knee. Alternate between bending the left and right knee in a controlled manner. Ensure a smooth transition between each leg movement, keeping a steady pace.

4. Continue alternating knee bends for the recommended number of repetitions. Focus on the straight leg's flexibility and the opposite knee's controlled bending.

Keep your palms on the floor for support throughout the exercise.

Full Body Rocking

Full body rocking is a holistic exercise that creates a seamless connection between your toes and head. By coordinating the movement of your feet and synchronizing it with your breath, this practice encourages a harmonious link throughout your entire body.

Here are the steps to practice this exercise:

1. Begin by lying on your back, spreading your legs wider than shoulder-width apart. Keep your arms next to your body, palms facing down.

2. Lift your toes up towards the ceiling, gently stretching your feet. Inhale deeply through your nose, allowing your lungs to fill with air. Hold the inhale comfortably, ideally between 3 to 5 seconds.

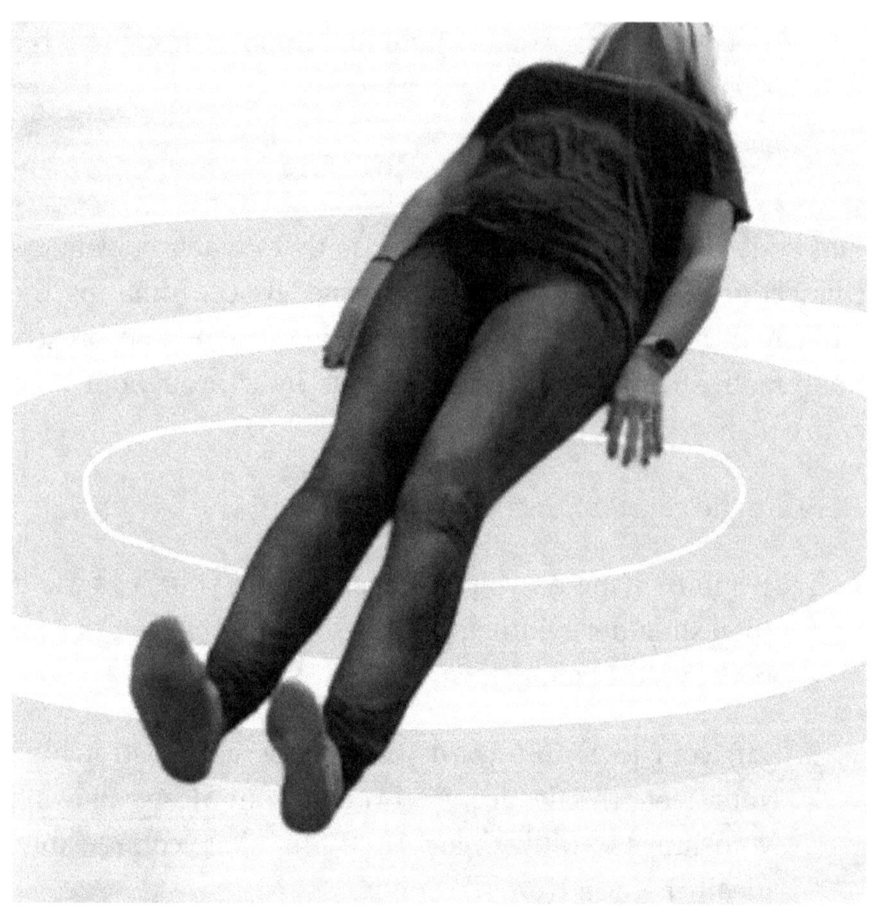

3. Extend your toes away from your body, pointing them as if reaching for the opposite end of the room. Exhale slowly and steadily through your mouth as if sipping through a straw. Hold the exhaled position for a relaxing duration, aiming for 5 to 8 seconds.

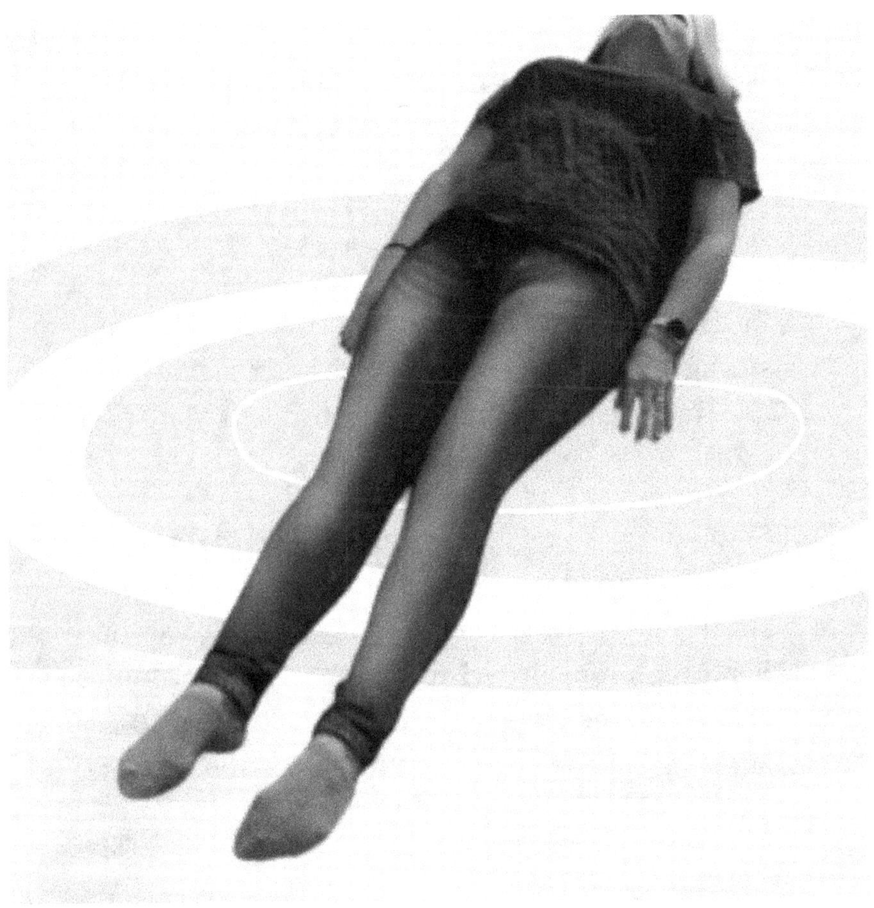

4. Return to the starting position, relaxing your toes and allowing them to spread naturally. Repeat the toe lift and inhale, followed by the toe stretch and exhale for the recommended number of repetitions.

Stretch and Compress

Stretch and Compress is a fantastic exercise designed to enhance mobility and relieve tension in your back. This position supports a healthy back and benefits your knees and ankles. Embracing these basic and natural postures comes with various advantages, particularly for those with sedentary lifestyles.

Here are the steps to practice this exercise:

1. Begin by sitting on the mat with your shins beneath you, sitting on your ankles. Extend your arms in front of you, creating a comfortable stretch through your back and arms.

2. Shift your body slightly to the left side, creating a lateral stretch. Extend your left arm to the left, feeling a gentle stretch along the left side of your torso. Place your right hand on your left wrist, adding a subtle compression element to the stretch. Hold this position for 10 seconds, allowing your body to settle into the stretch.

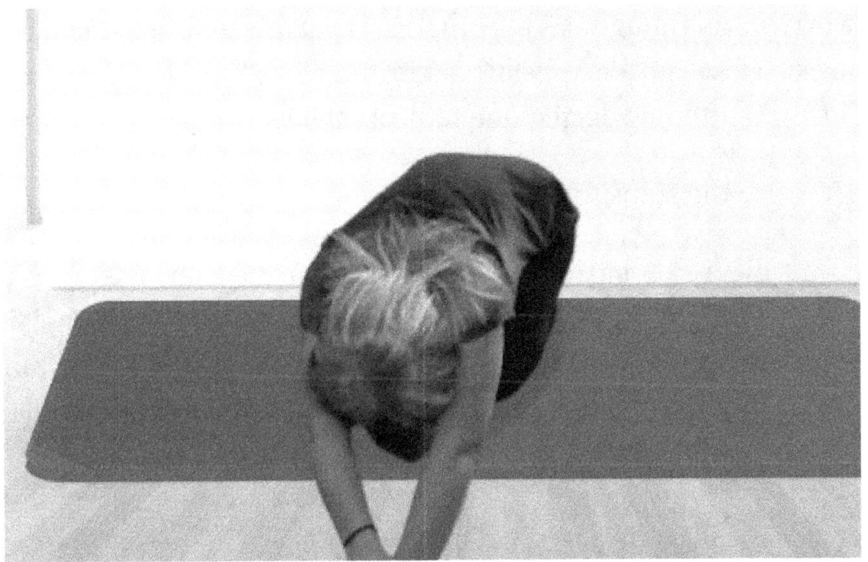

3. Return to the center and shift your body slightly to the right side. Extend your right arm slightly to the right with your left hand on top of your right wrist. Hold this mirrored position for another 10 seconds, feeling the stretch along the right side of your torso.

4. Slowly release the stretch and compression, returning to the center. Take a moment to notice any sensations and changes in your body. Repeat the exercise for the desired number of sets, focusing on the fluid movement and the balance between stretch and compression.

Energy Opening

Energy opening is a simple and beneficial exercise that promotes relaxation and mindfulness. By letting go of anxiety and concentrating on the present moment, it helps release worries and thoughts. This practice is particularly beneficial for neck, back, and knee health as it involves assuming a natural position often neglected due to prolonged sitting.

Here are the steps to practice this exercise:

1. Begin by sitting on your shins on the mat, ensuring a straight back. Place your hands behind your head, dropping your chin towards your collarbone. Keep your elbows closed, creating a centered and grounded starting position.

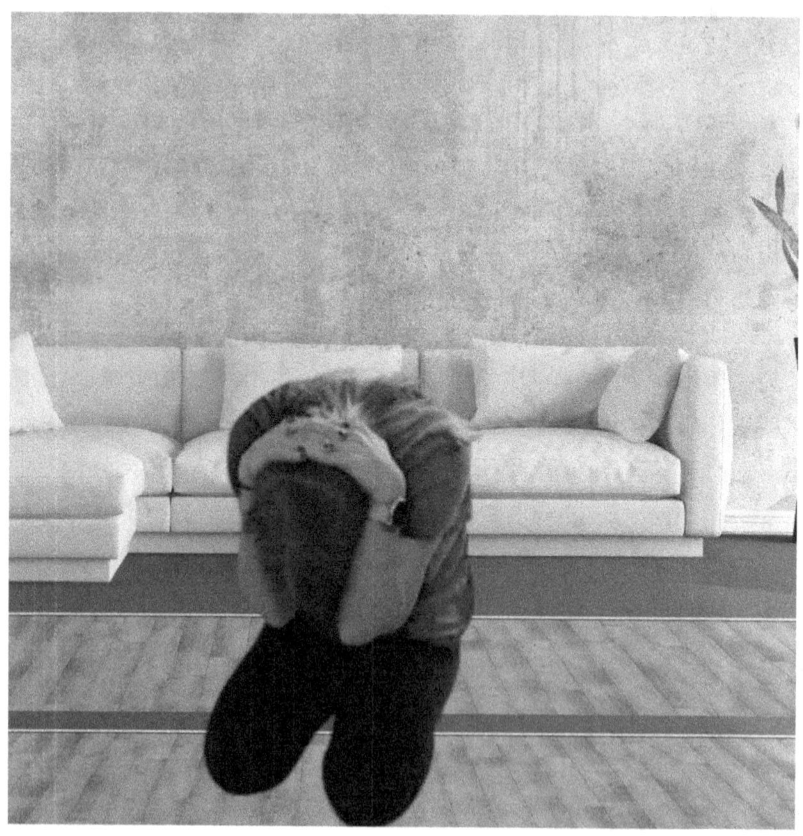

2. Inhale deeply, lifting your head while simultaneously exhaling. Open up your elbows and chest as you lift your head, creating a gentle arch in your upper body. Maintain your hands on the back of your head throughout this movement. As you continue to exhale, feel the expansion in your chest and the energy opening up in your upper body. Focus on the intentional opening of your elbows and the lift in your head.

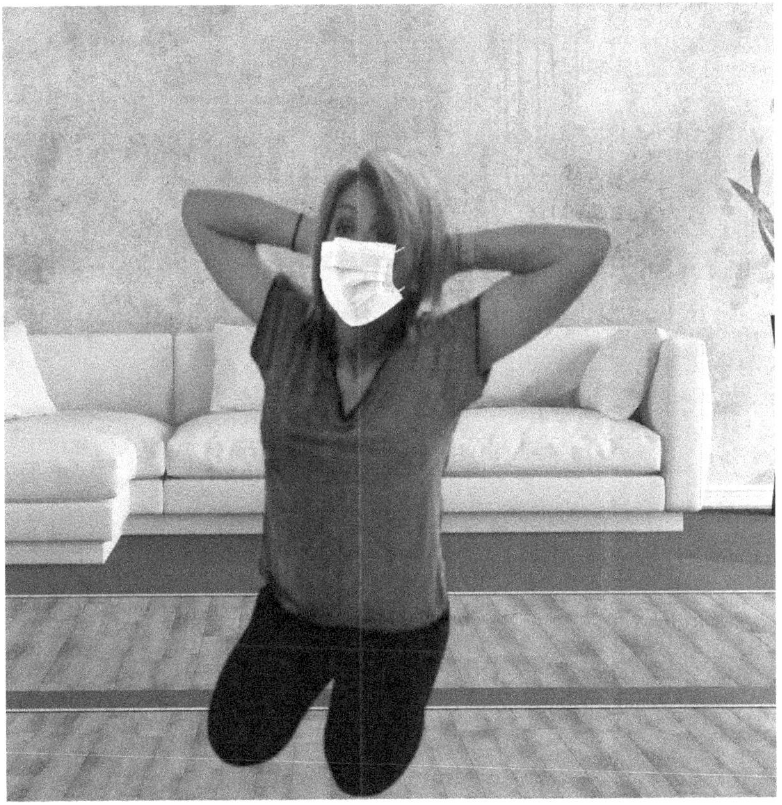

3. Exhale fully as you gracefully return to the initial step, lowering your head and closing your elbows. Keep your

movements controlled and synchronized with your breath.

4. Repeat the sequence for the desired number of repetitions. Pay attention to the flow of energy in your upper body and the sense of openness in your chest.

Knee Hold

The knee hold exercise is a fantastic way to boost coordination and balance while enhancing mobility in your lower body. By bringing your knee close to your chest, you not only engage your leg muscles but also find a sense of center and control over your body and emotions. Hugging your leg provides a comforting sensation and promotes positive emotions, helping to diminish negativity. Furthermore, this exercise strengthens your arms and upper body, offering a holistic benefit for physical and emotional well-being.

Here are the steps to practice this exercise:

1. Begin by standing on the mat, ensuring a stable and comfortable footing.

2. Lift one knee towards your chest, using both hands to gently bring it closer. Keep only one foot on the floor, allowing the lifted knee to reach toward your chest. Relax your whole body, emphasizing using your arms to guide the movement.

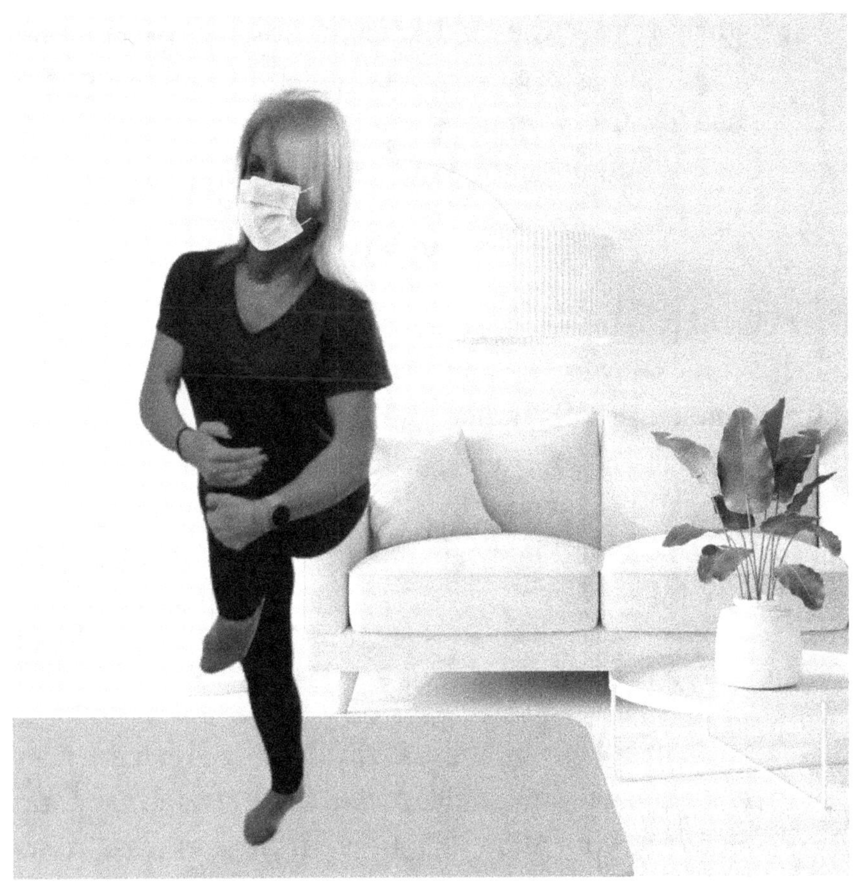

Focus on deep and controlled breathing throughout the exercise. Inhale slowly and deeply as you feel the stretch, and exhale gradually to promote relaxation. Keep your attention on your breath, allowing it to guide the rhythm of the movement.

3. Hold the knee close to your chest for 10 seconds. Continue breathing gently and maintain a relaxed posture. Feel the stretch in the lifted leg and the engagement in your arms.

4. Slowly release the held knee and return it to the mat. Repeat the exercise on the other leg, lifting the opposite knee towards your chest. Continue the sequence for the desired number of repetitions.

Open Life

The open life exercise is a wonderful way to boost your energy and happiness levels. It instills a sense of control over your body, enhancing both upper and lower body strength. This grounding exercise fosters a connection with your heart, promoting a deeper sense of well-being. As a bonus, open life improves posture and body alignment, contributing to overall physical health.

Here are the steps to practice this exercise:

1. Lie on your belly on the mat with your legs extended and relaxed. Keep your ankles relaxed, and stretch your arms out before you. Allow all muscles from your neck to your ankles to fully relax.

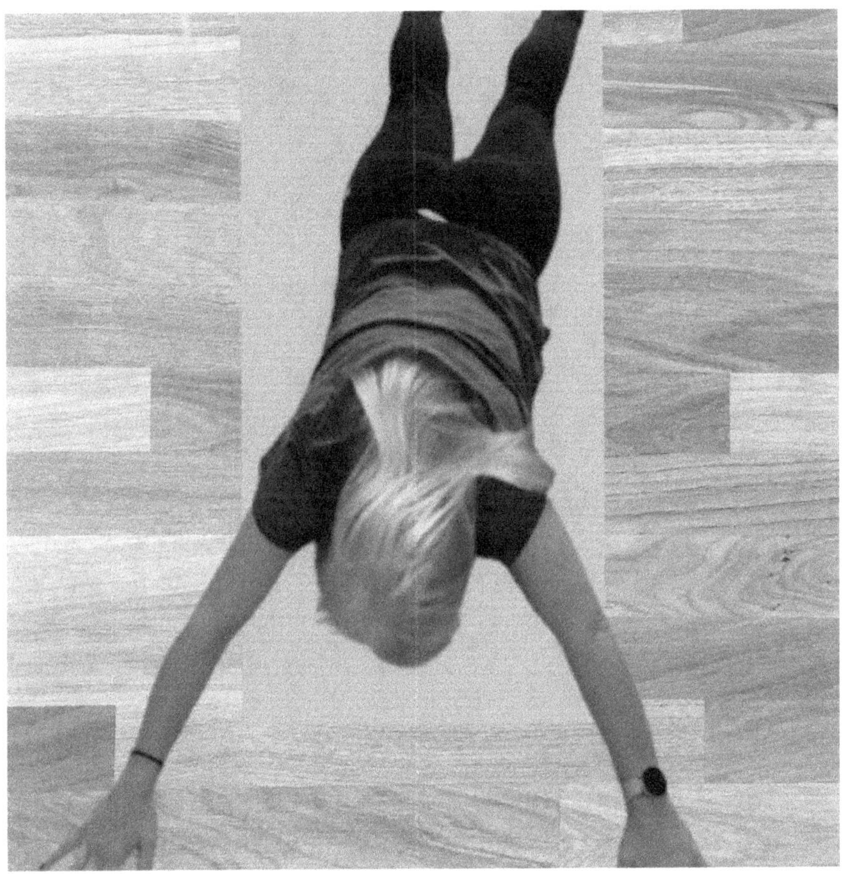

2. Inhale deeply and lift your arms and legs as much as possible, maintaining contact between your pelvis and core with the mat. Hold this lifted position for 2 seconds, focusing on the extension through your arms and legs. Feel the engagement in your back muscles and the stretch through your limbs.

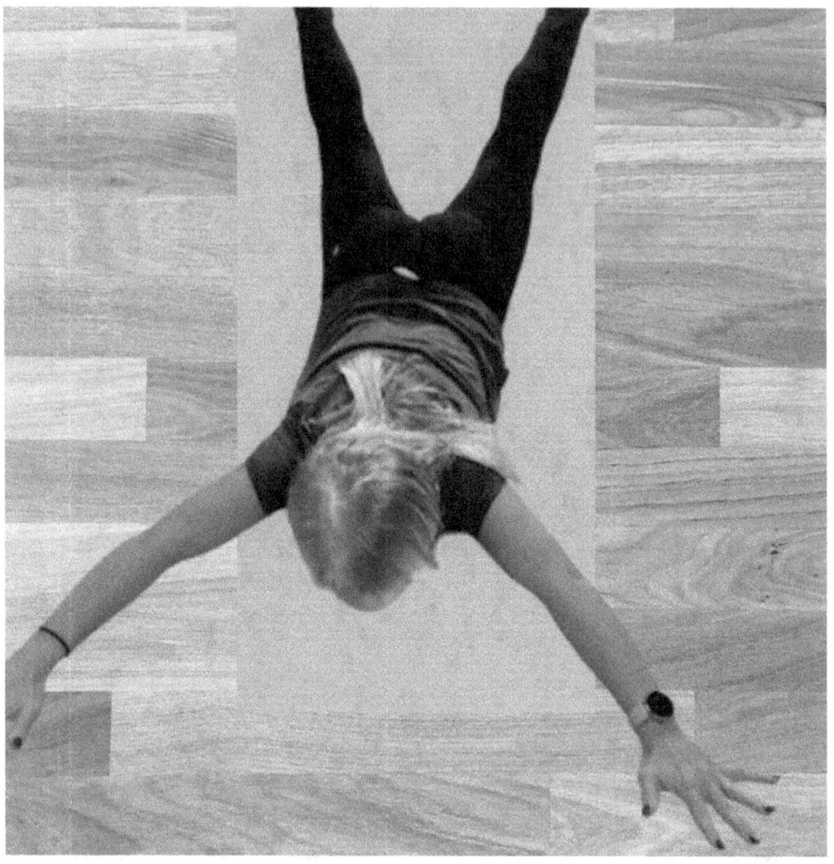

3. Exhale slowly and lower your arms and legs back to the starting position. Keep the movement controlled, ensuring a smooth return to the mat.

4. Perform the exercise for the specified number of repetitions. Focus on the inhale during the lift and the controlled exhale as you return to the starting position. Pay attention to the engagement in your back muscles and the overall sense of openness in your body.

Floor Star

The floor star exercise is crucial for getting ready for your workout or session. It's all about achieving a state of relaxation and connecting with your body. By taking deep breaths and consciously relaxing any tight or tense areas, you set a positive tone for your session. This exercise is recommended at the beginning of every session, ideally for at least ten deep breaths. Clear your mind of thoughts and worries, allowing yourself to focus on the present moment fully. This simple routine helps create a foundation for a more effective and mindful workout or activity.

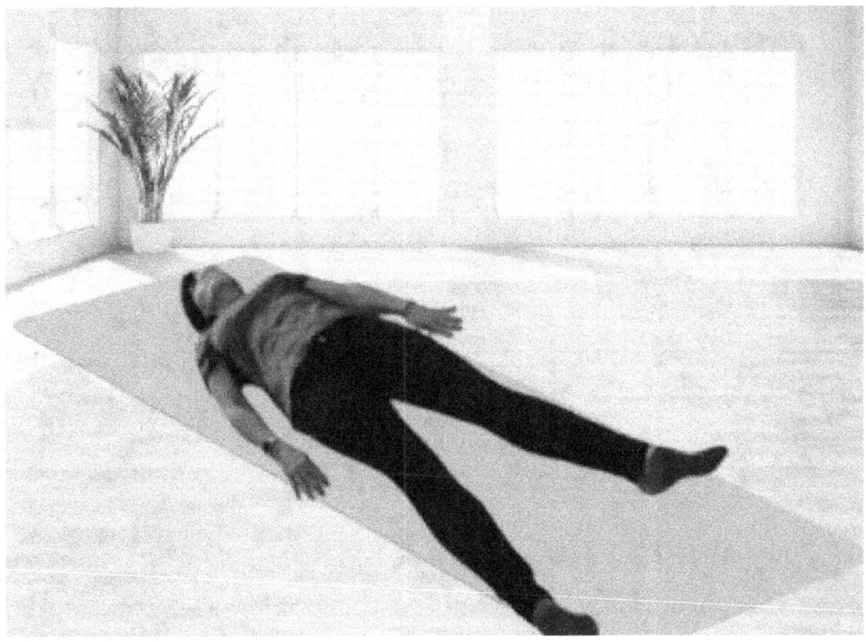

Here are the steps to practice this exercise:

1. Lie on your back with your legs spread wider than shoulder-width apart. Extend your arms to the sides of your body, creating an open and relaxed posture.

2. Concentrate on your breath, allowing it to become slow and rhythmic. Relax your entire body and be present in the moment, letting go of any tension or stress.

3. Pay attention to the parts of your body touching the mat, sensing any tension or tightness. Become aware of the natural curve of your spine, noting its alignment. Focus on your legs and find the most comfortable position for your feet, allowing them to settle naturally.

4. Inhale deeply through your nose, allowing your lungs to fill with air. Exhale through your mouth slowly and completely, releasing any residual tension. Repeat this deep breathing pattern at least ten times, fostering a sense of calm and relaxation.

5. If you feel particularly tense, feel free to extend the exercise for longer. Continue the deep breathing and mindfulness, allowing your body to unwind further.

Seated Forward Bend

The Seated Forward Bend, or Paschimottanasana in yoga, is a pose that brings various benefits to your overall well-being, including mental health. In this stretch, you sit with your legs extended and reach towards your toes. It helps to stretch and lengthen the spine, hamstrings, and lower back, promoting flexibility. The pose also encourages calmness and relaxation, making it beneficial for mental well-being by reducing stress and anxiety.

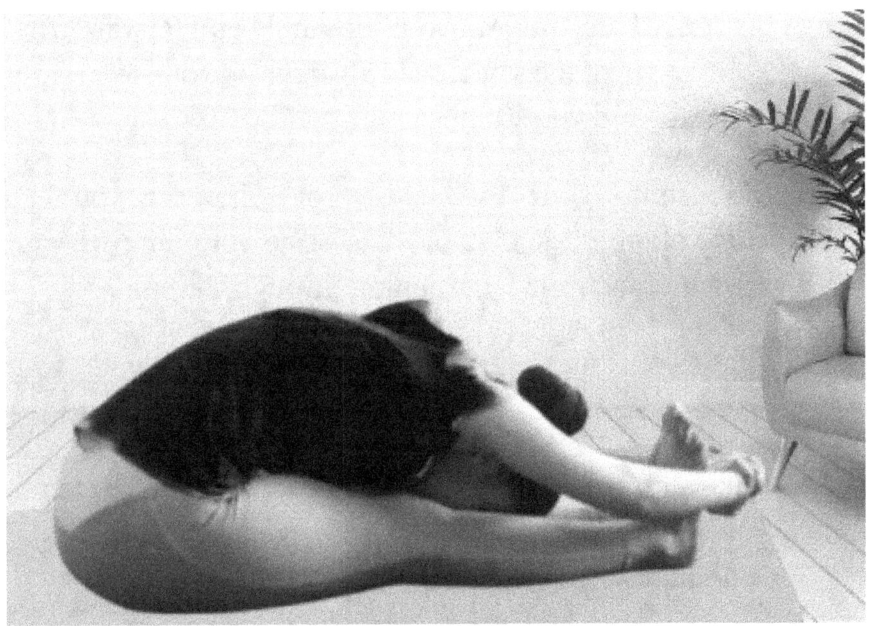

Here's how you can perform it:

1. Begin in a seated position on the floor with your legs extended straight in front of you. If needed, sit on a folded blanket or cushion for support, especially if you have tight hamstrings.

2. Sit tall, lengthening your spine. Engage your core muscles to provide support for your back.

3. Point your toes towards the ceiling, activating the muscles in your legs.

4. Inhale deeply as you raise your arms overhead. Lengthen your spine and reach toward the ceiling, emphasizing a gentle stretch.

5. As you exhale, hinge at your hips and bend forward from your waist. Keep your back straight as you lower your chest toward your thighs.

6. Hold onto your feet, shins, or wherever you can comfortably reach. Avoid excessive rounding of your back and focus on lengthening through the spine.

   Allow your head and neck to relax. Optionally, let your hands rest on your feet or the floor beside your legs.

7. Take slow, deep breaths in and out. Feel the stretch in your hamstrings and lower back, promoting a sense of calm and stress relief.

8. Stay in the forward fold for 30 seconds to a minute, gradually increasing the duration as you become more comfortable.

9. On an inhale, slowly lift your torso back to an upright position. Feel the lengthening of your spine as you return to the seated position.

Legs Up the Wall Pose

Legs up the Wall Pose is a soothing inverted yoga position that relieves the legs, feet, spine, and nervous system. By lying on your back and extending your legs up against a wall, you allow gravity to work in your favor, reducing strain on your lower body. This gentle pose promotes deep relaxation and rejuvenation, making it an excellent choice for stress relief. Legs up the Wall is known for its calming effects on the nervous system, making it a valuable practice for winding down and restoring the body after a busy day.

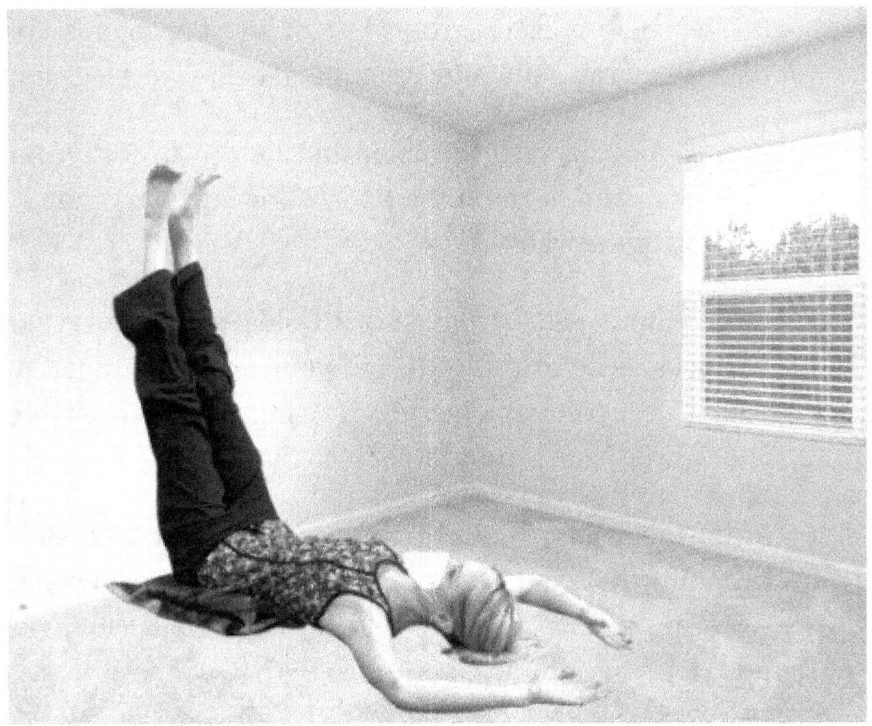

Here's how you can practice this exercise:

1. Set a bolster or a firm, long pillow on the floor against the wall. Ensure a comfortable space where you can easily sit with your left side against the wall.

2. Sit with your left side against the wall, ensuring your lower back rests against the bolster if you're using one. If using a bolster, position your lower back onto the support.

3. Turn your body to the left and bring your legs onto the wall. If using a bolster, shift your lower back onto the bolster before lifting your legs. Use your hands for balance as you shift your weight and bring your legs up.

4. Lower your back to the floor and lie down. Rest your shoulders and head on the floor, allowing your spine to align with the wall.

5. Shift your weight from side to side and scoot your buttocks close to the wall. Let your arms rest open at your sides, palms facing up. If using a bolster, ensure your lower back is fully supported by it.

6. Allow the heads of your thigh bones to release and relax, dropping toward the back of your pelvis. Close your eyes, fostering a sense of calm and introspection. Hold the pose for 5-10 minutes, breathing with awareness.

7. To release, slowly push yourself away from the wall. Slide your legs down to the right side, using your hands to help press yourself back up to a seated position.

High Knees

High knees are a physical exercise that focuses on working the lower body, but their benefits extend beyond just muscles. Engaging in high knees, where you lift your knees towards your chest while jogging in place, contributes to overall well-being. Regular participation in physical activities like high knees has positively affected mood, reduced stress, and improved cognitive function. So, while the primary target is your lower body muscles, exercise also promotes mental health and overall fitness.

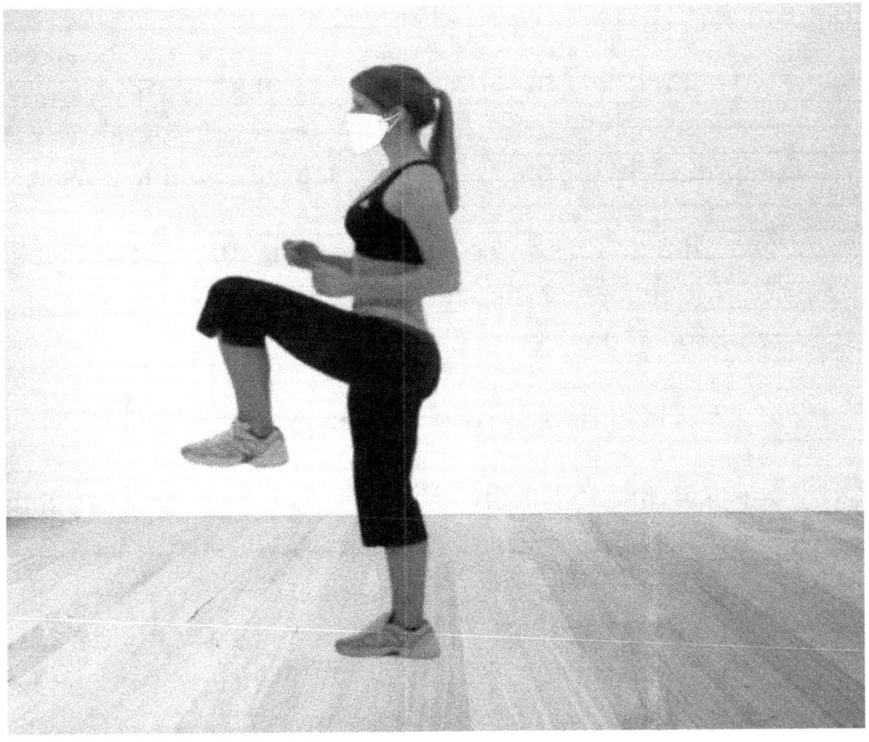

Here are the steps to practice this exercise:

1. Stand on a flat surface, ensuring a stable footing.

2. Start jogging in place, lifting your knees to a comfortable height. Focus on maintaining a steady and controlled pace.

3. Gradually lift your knees higher, aiming for hip level. Keep your core tight to provide support for your back during the movement.

4. For an advanced version, extend your arms straight at hip level. Try to touch your knees to your hands, maintaining a strong and engaged core.

5. Pay attention to bringing your knees towards your hands, avoiding reaching your hands to the knees. It emphasizes the engagement of your abdominal muscles.

6. Continue the exercise by repeating the above steps. Maintain a consistent rhythm and focus on the controlled movement of lifting your knees.

Overhead Side Reach Stretch

The Overhead Side Reach Stretch is a physical exercise focusing on the muscles in your torso, shoulders, and arms. You engage and stretch these muscle groups by reaching your arms overhead and leaning to the side. While physical activities like this stretch can positively affect overall well-being, it's essential to recognize that mental health is a multifaceted aspect of well-being. While the stretch contributes to flexibility and muscle toning, maintaining good mental health involves various factors such as a balanced lifestyle, social connections, and emotional well-being.

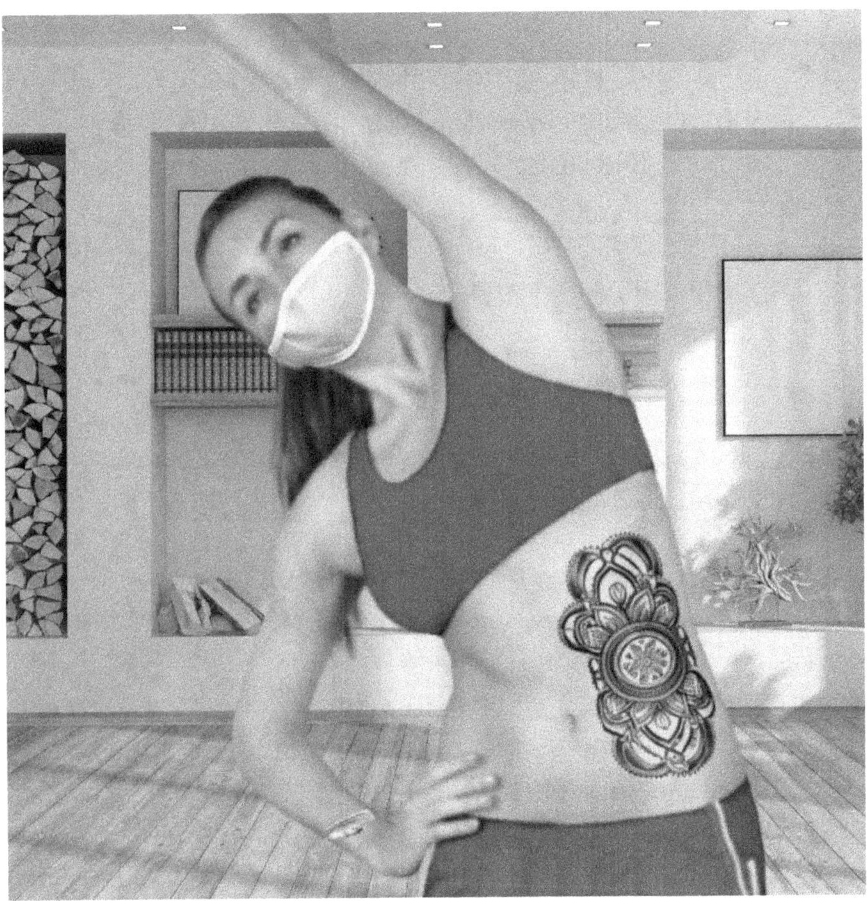

Here's how you can perform this exercise:

1. Stand tall with your feet about hip-width apart or slightly wider for better balance. Place your left hand at your side, with your palm touching your thigh.

2. Raise your right hand above your head, extending your elbow and shoulder fully. Point your fingertips toward the sky, feeling a gentle stretch along the right side of your torso.

3. Keep your right arm elevated and lean to the left. Lower your left hand along your thigh until you feel a comfortable stretch on the right side of your torso.

4. Allow your neck to drop and sink into the stretch, maintaining a relaxed posture. Feel the elongation along the entire right side of your body.

5. Stay in this stretched position for five to 10 seconds, focusing on the sensation of the stretch. Ensure you feel a gentle tug along the right side of your torso.

6. Gradually return to your starting position, standing tall with both arms by your sides.

7. Perform the same sequence on the other side, raising your left hand and leaning to the right. Feel the stretch along the left side of your torso.

8. Continue alternating between the left and right sides. Aim for 10 to 20 repetitions, completing two to three sets for a comprehensive stretch session.

Seated Torso Twist

The Seated Torso Twist is a yoga pose that offers several benefits for mental health. This pose helps promote relaxation, reduce stress, and increase mindfulness by gently twisting your upper body while seated. The gentle rotation engages the spine and encourages flexibility in the back muscles. Additionally, focusing on deep breathing during the twist enhances the mind-body connection, bringing a sense of calmness and mental clarity.

Here's how you can do it:

1. Sit on the floor with your legs extended in front of you. Ensure your back is straight, and engage your core for stability.

2. Cross your right leg over the other, placing your right foot flat on the floor in line with your left knee. Allow your knee to point towards the ceiling.

3. With your left arm, reach across and push against the outer side of your bent right knee. Simultaneously, twist your head slowly to the right, looking behind your shoulder. Feel the gentle twist along your spine.

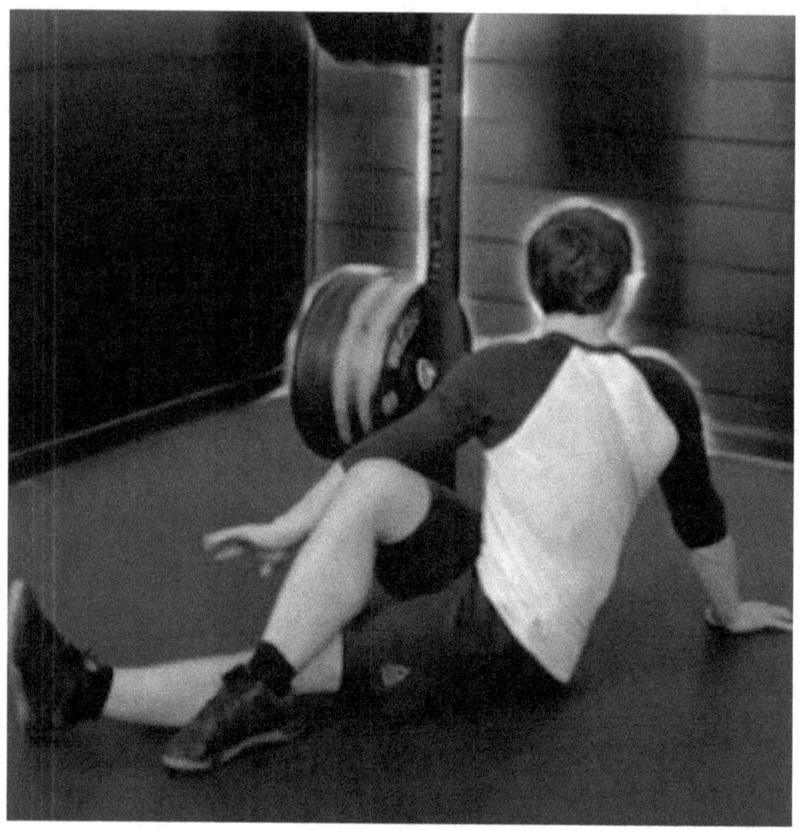

4. Hold the seated torso twist for 30 seconds, allowing your body to settle into the stretch. Focus on breathing deeply to enhance the stretch and promote relaxation.

5. Release the twist and return to the starting position. Uncross your legs and extend them out in front of you. Repeat the exercise on the other side by crossing your left leg over and twisting to the left.

CHAPTER 3: 28-DAY PLAN

Take a 28-day journey to improve your mental and physical well-being with my specially designed somatic exercise plan. These daily exercises offer more than just a physical workout—they provide a practical approach to overall wellness. By dedicating a few minutes each day to specific movements, you'll see positive changes in your flexibility, strength, and overall health.

Not only do these exercises have physical benefits, but they also promote a deeper connection between your body and mind. With simple breathing techniques, these exercises help relax tense muscles and calm the mind. By focusing on your breath during the routines, you can be more present in the moment and enhance your body awareness. This approach not only reduces stress and anxiety but also contributes to an improved appearance, reflecting the inner balance achieved through practice.

Note: Before starting the daily somatic exercises, you must perform 8-10 reps of full body rocking. It will help activate your muscles and joints, promoting flexibility and mobility throughout the body.

Day 1

Exercise	Repetitions
Neck Release	6 reps each side
Back Arch	6 reps
Hamstring Stretch	4 reps each side
Chest Opener	3 reps each side
Hip Flexor Stretch	6 reps
Baby Stretch	4 reps each side

Day 2

Exercise	Repetitions
Pelvic Preparation	4 reps
Moving Rock	6 reps
Despair	4 reps

Superman	6 reps
Side Reach	4 reps each side
Spinal Wave	6 reps
Reach Back	(4 reps each side

Day 3

Exercise	Repetitions
Standing Reach	4 reps
Spider Circle	6 reps
Star Glute Bridge	5 reps
Standing Stress Release	3 reps
Standing Spider	4 reps each side
Full Body Rocking	8 reps)

Day 4

Exercise	Repetitions
Stretch and Compress	4 reps each side
Energy Opening	6 reps
Knee Hold	4 reps
Open Life	5 reps
Floor Star	4 reps
Seated Forward Bend	6 reps

Day 5

Exercise	Repetitions
Legs Up the Wall Pose	4 reps

High Knees	6 reps
Overhead Side Reach Stretch	4 reps each side
Seated Torso Twist	6 reps
Neck Release	4 reps each side
Back Arch	6 reps
Hamstring Stretch	4 reps each side

Day 6

Exercise	Repetitions
Chest Opener	3 reps each side
Hip Flexor Stretch	6 reps
Baby Stretch	4 reps each side
Pelvic Preparation	4 reps

Moving Rock	6 reps
Despair	4 reps
Superman	6 reps

Day 7

Exercise	Repetitions
Side Reach	4 reps each side
Spinal Wave	6 reps
Reach Back	4 reps each side
Standing Reach	4 reps
Spider Circle	6 reps
Star Glute Bridge	5 reps
Standing Stress Release	3 reps

Day 8

Exercise	Repetitions
Standing Spider	4 reps each side
Full Body Rocking	8 reps
Stretch and Compress	4 reps each side
Energy Opening	6 reps
Knee Hold	4 reps
Open Life	5 reps
Floor Star	4 reps

Day 9

Exercise	Repetitions

Seated Forward Bend	6 reps
Legs Up the Wall Pose	4 reps
High Knees	6 reps
Overhead Side Reach Stretch	4 reps each side
Seated Torso Twist	6 reps
Neck Release	4 reps each side
Back Arch	6 reps

Day 10

Exercise	Repetitions
Hamstring Stretch	4 reps each side
Chest Opener	3 reps each side
Hip Flexor Stretch	6 reps

Baby Stretch	4 reps each side
Pelvic Preparation	4 reps
Moving Rock	6 reps
Despair	4 reps

Day 11

Exercise	Repetitions
Superman	6 reps
Side Reach	4 reps each side
Spinal Wave	6 reps
Reach Back	4 reps each side
Standing Reach	4 reps
Spider Circle	6 reps

Star Glute Bridge	5 reps

Day 12

Exercise	Repetitions
Standing Stress Release	3 reps
Standing Spider	4 reps each side
Full Body Rocking	8 reps
Stretch and Compress	4 reps each side
Energy Opening	6 reps
Knee Hold	4 reps

Day 13

Exercise	Repetitions

Open Life	5 reps
Floor Star	4 reps
Seated Forward Bend	6 reps
Legs Up the Wall Pose	4 reps
High Knees	6 reps
Overhead Side Reach Stretch	4 reps each side

Day 14

Exercise	Repetitions
Seated Torso Twist	6 reps
Neck Release	4 reps each side
Back Arch	6 reps
Hamstring Stretch	4 reps each side

Chest Opener	3 reps each side
Hip Flexor Stretch	6 reps
Baby Stretch	4 reps each side

Day 15

Exercise	Repetitions
Pelvic Preparation	4 reps
Moving Rock	6 reps
Despair	4 reps
Superman	6 reps
Side Reach	4 reps each side
Spinal Wave	6 reps
Reach Back	4 reps each side

Day 16

Exercise	Repetitions
Standing Reach	4 reps
Spider Circle	6 reps
Star Glute Bridge	5 reps
Standing Stress Release	3 reps
Standing Spider	4 reps each side
Full Body Rocking	8 reps

Day 17

Exercise	Repetitions
Stretch and Compress	4 reps each side

Energy Opening	6 reps
Knee Hold	4 reps
Open Life	5 reps
Floor Star	4 reps
Seated Forward Bend	6 reps

Day 18

Exercise	Repetitions
Legs Up the Wall Pose	4 reps
High Knees	6 reps
Overhead Side Reach Stretch	4 reps each side
Seated Torso Twist	6 reps
Neck Release	4 reps each side

Back Arch	6 reps
Hamstring Stretch	4 reps each side

Day 19

Exercise	Repetitions
Chest Opener	3 reps each side
Hip Flexor Stretch	6 reps
Baby Stretch	4 reps each side
Pelvic Preparation	4 reps
Moving Rock	6 reps
Despair	4reps
Superman	6 reps

Day 20

Exercise	Repetitions
Side Reach	4 reps each side
Spinal Wave	6 reps
Reach Back	4 reps each side
Standing Reach	4 reps
Spider Circle	6 reps
Star Glute Bridge	5 reps
Standing Stress Release	3 reps

Day 21

Exercise	Repetitions
Standing Spider	4 reps each side
Full Body Rocking	8 reps

Stretch and Compress	4 reps each side
Energy Opening	6 reps
Knee Hold	4 reps
Open Life	5 reps
Floor Star	4 reps

Day 22

Exercise	Repetitions
Seated Torso Twist	6 reps
Neck Release	4 reps each side
Back Arch	6 reps
Hamstring Stretch	4 reps each side
Chest Opener	3 reps each side

Hip Flexor Stretch	6 reps
Baby Stretch	4 reps each side

Day 23

Exercise	Repetitions
Hamstring Stretch	4 reps each side
Chest Opener	3 reps each side
Hip Flexor Stretch	6 reps
Baby Stretch	4 reps each side
Pelvic Preparation	4 reps
Moving Rock	6 reps
Despair	4 reps

Day 24

Exercise	Repetitions
Superman	6 reps
Side Reach	4 reps each side
Spinal Wave	6 reps
Reach Back	4 reps each side
Standing Reach	4 reps
Spider Circle	6 reps
Star Glute Bridge	5 reps

Day 25

Exercise	Repetitions
Standing Stress Release	3 reps
Standing Spider	4 reps each side

Full Body Rocking	8 reps
Stretch and Compress	4 reps each side
Energy Opening	6 reps
Knee Hold	4 reps

Day 26

Exercise	Repetitions
Standing Reach	4 reps
Spider Circle	4 reps
Star Glute Bridge	4 reps
Standing Stress Release	4 reps
Standing Spider	4 reps each side alternated
Full Body Rocking	5 reps

Stretch and Compress	4 reps

Day 27

Exercise	Repetitions
Energy Opening	4 reps
Knee Hold	4 reps
Open Life	4 reps
Floor Star	4 reps
Seated Forward Bend	4 reps
Legs Up the Wall Pose	4 reps
High Knees	4 reps

Day 28

Exercise	Repetitions
Pelvic Preparation	4 reps
Moving Rock	6 reps
Despair	4 reps
Superman	6 reps
Side Reach	4 reps each side
Spinal Wave	6 reps
Reach Back	4 reps each side

CONCLUSION

Starting somatic exercises is an empowering step towards cultivating a harmonious connection between the mind and body. This book serves as a comprehensive guide for beginners, offering a clear understanding of somatics and presenting a variety of exercises with accompanying images for easy implementation.

I explored the essence of somatic exercises, delving into their transformative potential for enhancing body awareness, relieving tension, and promoting overall well-being. By breaking down various somatic exercises in simple terms, accompanied by visual aids, I aimed to make the learning process accessible and enjoyable for readers of all levels.

The 28-day plan outlined in this book provides a structured approach for those eager to incorporate somatic exercises into their daily routine. Through consistent practice, readers can cultivate mindfulness, release muscular tension, and foster a deeper connection with their bodies.

•